Real-Time
Three-Dimensional
Transesophageal
Echocardiography

Annette Vegas • Massimiliano Meineri
Angela Jerath

Real-Time Three-Dimensional Transesophageal Echocardiography

A Step-by-Step Guide

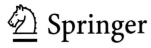 Springer

Annette Vegas, MD, FRCPC, FASE
Associate Professor of Anesthesiology
Director of Perioperative TEE

Massimiliano Meineri, MD
Assistant Professor of Anesthesiology

Angela Jerath, FRCPC, FANZCA, BSc, MBBS
Assistant Professor of Anesthesiology

Department of Anesthesia
Toronto General Hospital
University of Toronto
Toronto, Ontario
M5G 2C4
Canada

ISBN 978-1-4614-0664-8   e-ISBN 978-1-4614-0665-5
DOI 10.1007/978-1-4614-0665-5
Springer New York Dordrecht Heidelberg London

Library of Congress Control Number: 2011933838

© Springer Science+Business Media, LLC 2012
All rights reserved. This work may not be translated or copied in whole or in part without the written permission of the publisher (Springer Science+Business Media, LLC, 233 Spring Street, New York, NY 10013, USA), except for brief excerpts in connection with reviews or scholarly analysis. Use in connection with any form of information storage and retrieval, electronic adaptation, computer software, or by similar or dissimilar methodology now known or hereafter developed is forbidden.
The use in this publication of trade names, trademarks, service marks, and similar terms, even if they are not identified as such, is not to be taken as an expression of opinion as to whether or not they are subject to proprietary rights. While the advice and information in this book are believed to be true and accurate at the date of going to press, neither the authors nor the editors nor the publisher can accept any legal responsibility for any errors or omissions that may be made. The publisher makes no warranty, express or implied, with respect to the material contained herein.

Printed on acid-free paper

Springer is part of Springer Science+Business Media (www.springer.com/mycopy)

Dedications

Annette Vegas

To my mentors, Dr DCH Cheng, Dr Andre Denault, Dr Harry Rakowski, and Dr Susan Lenkei, for their unwavering support and believing in my dreams

Massimilliano Meineri

To Rosa Maria for her continuous unconditioned support and constant inspiration

Angela Jerath

To the pure continuum and Words of Zohra and Santosh

Preface

Three-dimensional (3D) transesophageal echocardiography (TEE) is a potent visual medium which can be used by the novice or experienced echocardiographer, cardiologist, and cardiac surgeon. It can achieve a better understanding and assessment of normal and pathological cardiac function and anatomy. This new technology complements traditional 2D imaging and permits visualization of any cardiac structure of interest from multiple perspectives. 3D technology challenges the echocardiographer to acquire a different skill set for image acquisition and manipulation.

This handbook is created in response to a need for a succinct illustrative synopsis on 3D technology and image acquisition. We have aimed to provide a simple step-by-step guide to the practical fundamentals of this technology, altered knobology, and how to acquire and manipulate image datasets. The chapters encompass normal and common cardiac pathology. As with all written echocardiography texts, still 3D images do not do justice to the cardiac activity seen in a live video clip. Hence, we advise readers to refer to other video sources including the TEE Perioperative Interactive Education (PIE) Web site, http://pie.med.utoronto.ca/TEE, which provides a wealth of free on-line video material.

This handbook is a compilation of echocardiography information and perioperative TEE images performed at Toronto General Hospital (TGH), Toronto, Ontario, Canada. The images are unaltered except for cropping to fit the size of the book. All 3D TEE images were acquired using an Ie33 machine and X7-2t 3D TEE probe (Philips Medical System, Andover, Massachusetts, USA). None of the authors have received any financial support from the industry during this project. At the time of writing, this monograph represents the current technology in this field based predominantly on this single vendor. Growth in this field continues as evidenced by technological advances and an increasing number of publications.

Dr. Annette Vegas
Dr. Massimilliano Meineri
Dr. Angela Jerath
April 2011

Acknowledgments

To members of the current TGH Anesthesiology Perioperative TEE group: Drs. L. Bahrey, G. Djaiani, J. Heggie, M. Jariani, J. Karski, R. Katznelson, P. McNama, P. Murphy, P. Slinger, A. Van Rensburg, and M. Wasowicz, who perform, train, and educate others about TEE.

To our colleagues from the Division of Cardiac Surgery, under the leadership of Dr. Tirone E. David, who attract a varied practice that keeps TGH cardiac anesthesiologists challenged to provide exemplary patient care.

To members of the TGH cardiology echocardiography lab, under the direction of Dr. Anna Woo and former directors Dr. Sam Siu and Dr. Harry Rakowski, who generously share their knowledge with the perioperative TEE group at TGH.

To medical student Mr. Gian-Marco Busato, MSc, for his extraordinary artistic talent he used to draw the illustrations for this handbook.

Finally to Ms. Willa Bradshaw, BSc, MScBMC, and Ms. Frances Yeung, BSc, MScBMC, medical illustrators, who precisely assembled all the detailed figures.

Contents

Abbreviations

A	Anterior
AC	Anterior commissure
ACB	Aortocoronary bypass
AHA	American Heart Association
AI	Aortic insufficiency
AL	Anterolateral
AMVL	Anterior mitral valve leaflet
AS	Aortic stenosis
ASD	Atrial septal defect
ASE	American Society of Echocardiography
AV	Aortic valve
AVA	Aortic valve area
AVR	Aortic valve replacement
BAV	Bicuspid aortic valve
BPM	Beats per minute
C	Chamber
CAD	Coronary artery disease
CE	Carpentier-Edwards
CO	Cardiac output
CPB	Cardiopulmonary bypass
CS	Coronary sinus
CSA	Cross-sectional area
CVP	Central venous pressure
CW	Continuous wave
ECG	Electrocardiogram
ED	End-diastole
EDA	End-diastolic area
EDD	End-diastolic diameter
EDV	End-diastolic volume
EF	Ejection fraction

Abbreviations

EI	Eccentricity index
ERO	Effective regurgitant orifice
ES	End-systole
ESA	End-systolic area
ESD	End-systolic diameter
ESV	End-systolic volume
FAC	Fractional area change
FL	False lumen
FR	Frame rate
FS	Fractional shortening
FV	Full volume
GE	Gastroesophageal
HBP	High blood pressure
HOCM	Hypertrophic obstructive cardiomyopathy
HR	Heart rate
HV	Hepatic vein
HVR	High volume rate
I	Inferior
IABP	Intra-aortic balloon pump
IAS	Inter-atrial septum
IHSS	Idiopathic hypertrophic subaortic stenosis
ITD	Intertrigonal distance
IVC	Inferior vena cava
IVV	Isovolumetric contraction
IVS	Interventricular septum
JA	Jet area
JH	Jet height
L	Left or lateral or length
LAA	Left atrial appendage
LA	Left atrium
LAE	Left atrial enlargement
LAP	Left atrial pressure
LAX	Long axis
LCA	Left coronary artery
LCC	Left coronary cusp
LMA	Left main coronary artery
LLPV	Left lower pulmonary vein
LSA	Left subclavian artery
LUPV	Left upper pulmonary vein

Abbreviations

LV	Left ventricle
LVAD	Left ventricular assist device
LVH	Left ventricular hypertrophy
LVID	Left ventricle internal diameter
LVOT	Left ventricular outflow tract
MAC	Mitral annular calcification
MC	Mitral commissural
ME	Midesophageal
MI	Myocardial infarction
MPR	Multiplanar reconstruction
MR	Mitral regurgitation
MS	Mitral stenosis
MV	Mitral valve
MVA	Mitral valve area
MVP	Mitral valve prolapse
MVQ	Mitral valve quantification
MVR	Mitral valve replacement
N	Non
NCC	Noncoronary cusp
NSR	Normal sinus rhythm
P	Pressure or posterior
PA	Pulmonary artery
PAP	Pulmonary artery pressure
PAPVD	Partial anomalous pulmonary venous drainage
PASP	Pulmonary artery systolic pressure
PC	Posterior commissure
PDA	Patent ductus arteriosus
PFO	Patent foramen ovale
PG	Pressure gradient
PHT	Pressure half-time
PI	Pulmonic insufficiency
PISA	Proximal isovelocity surface area
PM	Papillary muscles or posteromedial
PMVL	Posterior mitral valve leaflet
PS	Pulmonic stenosis
PV	Pulmonic valve
PVC	Premature ventricular contraction

Abbreviations

PW	Pulsed wave
PWT	Posterior wall thickness
R	Right
RA	Right atrium
RAP	Right atrial pressure
RCA	Right coronary artery
RCC	Right coronary cusp
RF	Regurgitant fraction
RLPV	Right lower pulmonary vein
ROI	Region of interest
RPA	Right pulmonary artery
RT	Real-time
RUPV	Right upper pulmonary vein
RV	Right ventricle
RVAD	Right ventricular assist device
RegV	Regurgitant volume
RVH	Right ventricular hypertrophy
RVOT	Right ventricular outflow tract
RVSP	Right ventricular systolic pressure
SAM	Systolic anterior motion
SAX	Short axis
SBP	Systolic blood pressure
SCA	Society of Cardiovascular Anesthesiology
SDI	Systolic dysynchrony index
STJ	Sinotubular junction
SV	Stroke volume
SVC	Superior vena cava
SVR	Systemic vascular resistance
SWMA	Segmental wall motion abnormality
SWT	Septal wall thickness
TAPSE	Tricuspid annular plane systolic excursion
TAV	Tricuspid annulus velocity
TDI	Tissue Doppler imaging
TEE	Transesophageal echocardiography
TG	Transgastric
TL	True lumen
TOF	Tetralogy of Fallot
TGA	Transposition of the great arteries
TMSV	Time to minimum systolic volume

Abbreviations

TR	Tricuspid regurgitation
TS	Tricuspid stenosis
TTE	Transthoracic echocardiography
TV	Tricuspid valve
TVA	Tricuspid valve area
UE	Upper esophageal
US	Ultrasound
VC	Vena contracta
VSD	Ventricular septal defect
VTI	Velocity time integral
2D	Two-dimensional
3D	Three-dimensional

1

Technology and 3D Imaging

A. Vegas et al., *Real-Time Three-Dimensional Transesophageal Echocardiography*, DOI 10.1007/978-1-4614-0665-5_1, © Springer Science+Business Media, LLC 2012

Introduction
Technology

The evolution of 3D echocardiography has been slow as it has involved time-consuming acquisition, off-line reconstruction and poor image quality. (A) Recent technological advances permit real-time (RT) 3D images using matrix array transducers that involve four steps: data acquisition, data storage, data processing and image display. Unlike standard 2D TEE imaging planes, 3D TEE relies on volume datasets. (B) Data processing, a 2-step process, transforms the scanned raw data in an ultrasound machine's computer RAM into a 3D dataset comprised of voxels. A voxel is a (vo)lume of pi(xels) used for display that describes the physical characteristics and location of the smallest cube in a dataset. Conversion places the raw data (white voxels) into a Cartesian volume with each assigned x-y-z coordinates and an echo-intensity value. Interpolation fills the gaps between all the known points in space with data points of similar characteristics (purple voxels). (C-E) 3D display is the 2-step process of making a 3D dataset visible, as either multiple 2D image planes or a 3D graphic reproduction. Segmentation separates within the 3D dataset the object to be rendered from surrounding structures. Increasingly complex rendering techniques create a visible 3D object from the same 3D dataset: wireframe, surface or volume rendering.

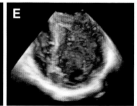

Image courtesy M. Corrin

(C) Wireframe rendering connects equidistant points on the 3D object surface with lines (wires) creating a mesh of small polygonal tiles. It is used for relatively flat surface structures such as the LV and the atrial cavities. (D) Surface rendering defines more points on the 3D object surface making the lines joining them invisible. It generates 3D objects with detailed surfaces and a hollow core. (E) Volume rendering displays a 3D object with a detailed surface and inner structure. The display of every voxel of the 3D object allows a "virtual dissection."

3D Echocardiographic Imaging

Volume Scanning

- Data Acquisition
  - Matrix Array Probe
  - TTE / TEE
- Data Storage
  - Computer RAM
- Data Processing
  - Conversion & Interpolation
  - 3D Graphic Rendering
- Data Display
  - Segmentation
  - Wire Frame | Surface Rendering | Volume Rendering

Raw Data

3D Volume Dataset

3D Image Display

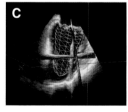

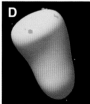

Introduction
Probes

(A) TTE and (B) TEE 3D probes contain matrix array transducers with 2,500 elements each of which is independently steered and focused. The stationary matrix array probe steers the ultrasound beam to scan and display (C) a pyramidal-shaped volume as compared with (D) the sector scan of a standard 2D TEE probe. Rapid 3D imaging occurs instantaneously over a single heartbeat or gated to multiple (4-7) heartbeats. Real time (RT) now defines any change of the displayed 3D image with probe movement. Compared to older technology, current gated 3D acquisitions are technically not RT but they practically are due to their near instantaneous display.

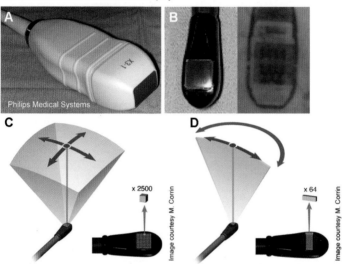

In most RT 3D modes, the reconstruction of intracardiac structures by volume rendering displays a pyramidal 3D dataset that can be rotated in any direction or cropped in any plane. The echocardiographer must attain new basic skills to acquire and manipulate the 3D datasets to an adequate orientation to show appropriate anatomy (see pg. 18). 3D Zoom of mitral valve with A1 and P1 prolapse is shown from (E) left atrium, (F) cropped at red line, (G) cropped and rotated sagittal views.

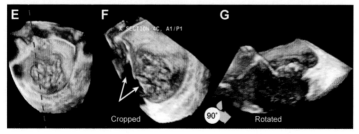

Introduction
2D Images

The 3D TEE matrix transducer (X7-2t, Philips Medical Systems, Andover, Massachusetts) functions as a standard 2D multiplane TEE probe including (A) 2D, (B) color, and (C) spectral Doppler modes. Tissue Doppler is only available with updated machine software. Sequential (phased) activation of individual crystals generates an ultrasound beam that is steered back and forth over a 90° angle to sweep a flat, "pie shaped" scanning plane or sector. Spectral Doppler and simple linear measurements are currently not possible in 3D modes, (D) but can be easily performed in 2D. Thus, RT 3D imaging complements but does not replace standard 2D TEE imaging.

Quality 3D images always start with a good 2D image. Any 2D artifact will persist in 3D.

1. Choose the best transducer frequency: resolution (high) > general (mid) > penetration (low). Harmonics improve 2D but not always 3D image quality.
2. Adjust the 2D overall gain and compression or use the time gain compensation (TGC) sliders. Single button 2D optimization may be available on the US machine.
3. Manipulate the 3D TEE probe to ensure good surface contact of the square transducer footprint to avoid distortion at the image edges. Further optimization of the dataset is required as described in pg. 20.

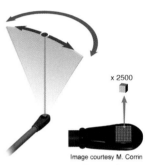

x 2500

Image courtesy M. Corrin

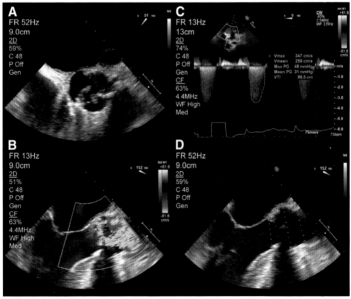

Introduction
xPlane

xPlane mode using the 3D TEE matrix transducer simultaneously displays 2 different 2D image planes with good spatial and temporal resolution (FR 30–40 Hz). The base image on the left display (blue plane A–C) and a second plane on the right display (red plane A–C) are obtained. The relationship between the images is shown by the angles in the circle. The solid line transducer angle is the base image, shown here is the (D) TG mid SAX 0° and (E) ME AV LAX 130°. The image on the right can be 90° to the base image (A, D) TG 2C, (B) adjusted to any multiplane angle or (C, E) obtained by moving a cursor line ME AV SAX –8°. (E) Color Doppler in xPlane mode has poor temporal resolution from an extremely low frame rate (FR 6 Hz).

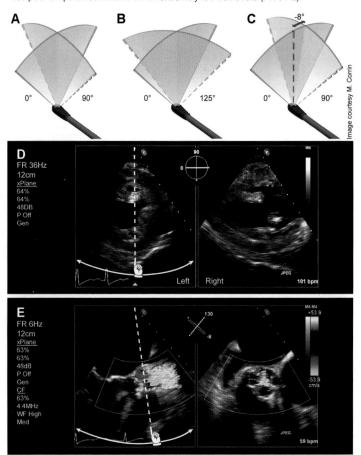

Introduction
3D Imaging Modes

Single button activation occurs for specific 3D imaging modes (ie33, Philips Medical Systems, Andover, Massachusetts) using matrix array probes. Choosing between modes for specific clinical applications is a balance between selecting pyramidal image size, frame rate (FR) and real-time (RT) imaging. 3D echocardiography has a complex relationship of FR, sector size, and image resolution interdependence. A change in one of these three factors alters the other two. Newer software allows independent manipulation of spatial resolution (image quality) and temporal resolution (FR) by acquiring images over multiple triggered heartbeats (see pg. 14).

3D imaging modes	Live (A)	Zoom (B)	Full Volume (C)
Dimensions (width × thickness × depth)	60° × 30° by 2D image depth	20° × 20° to 90° × 90° by variable height	90° × 90° by 2D image depth
Real time	Yes	Yes	No (gated)
Frame rate	20 - 30 Hz	5 - 20 Hz	20 - 40 Hz
Temporal resolution	Good	Low	Good
Spatial resolution	Mid	High	High
Cardiac structure	Any 2D image	Valves, IAS, LAA	MV, LV
Clinical applications	Guide interventions	Examine anatomy Guide interventions	LV function Color Doppler

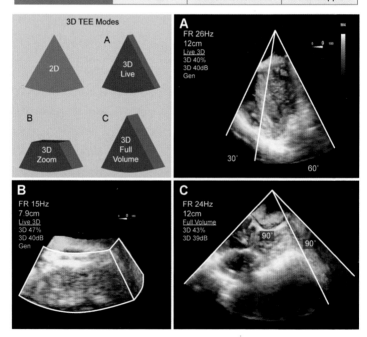

Introduction
Line Density and Frequency

Important determinants of 3D image quality and size are line density and transducer frequency. (A) Select low density if a wider sector is required to include the entire region of interest as for 3D color Doppler or full volume (FV), as shown in this base of the heart view. (B) High line density shows a smaller 3D image size but with better spatial resolution in all 3D imaging modes. The default for most modes is a medium line density. Transducer frequency is determined by the selection of options such as (C) penetration (low frequency), (D) general (intermediate frequency) or (F) resolution (high frequency) and like for 2D they can dramatically affect the image appearance.

Line density	Low	Medium	High
Live 3D	NA	58° × 29°	46° × 23°
3D Zoom	45° × 45°	38° × 38°	30° × 30°
Full Volume	93° × 84°	78° × 70°	62° × 56°
3D color	42° × 42°	35° × 35°	28° × 28°

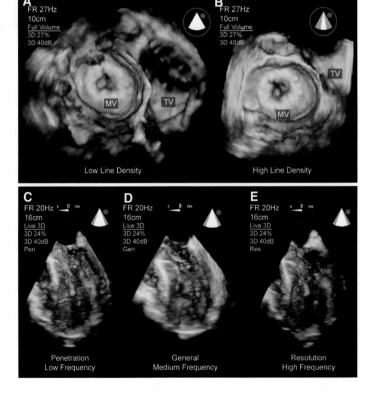

Introduction
Live 3D

Live 3D mode allows RT imaging with depth (perspective). Standard ME 4C views are obtained as (A) thin slices (90° × 1°) or (B) by default as a thicker segment (60° × 30°) with older software. The limited sector size necessitates physical probe movement to image entire structures. (C) High line density improves spatial resolution but with a smaller image size and similar FR, as shown for ME AV LAX views. Temporal resolution is adequate with FR 20–30 Hz. This mode is valuable as rotation of any 3D volume in RT can quickly check and be used to actively optimize 3D settings.

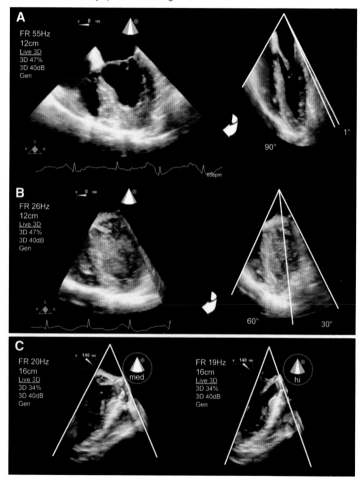

Introduction
Live 3D

Lateral steer overcomes sector size limitations without moving the probe. Moving the sector to the right or left will center the image structures. 3D Live ME 4C view (middle) is shown with TV and LV cut off. (A) Lateral steer (left) shows the entire TV annulus and RV. (B) Lateral steer (right) displays both LV walls and half of LV cavity.

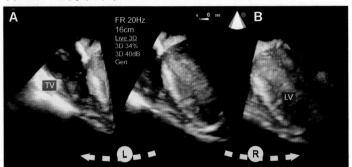

(C–E) The same aortic arch at 0° is shown using different imaging modes. A (C) standard 2D image of the UE Aortic Arch LAX view; (D) is the same plane obtained with the 3D Live mode, and (E) is a slightly tilted downwards (arrow) 3D Live dataset of (D) to view the intimal surface. These 3D images demonstrate better detail of the vessel intimal surface and can help determine the exact size and location of pathology. The near field remains difficult to see in both 2D and 3D TEE.

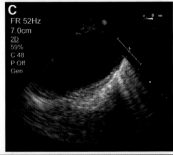

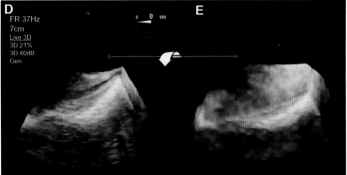

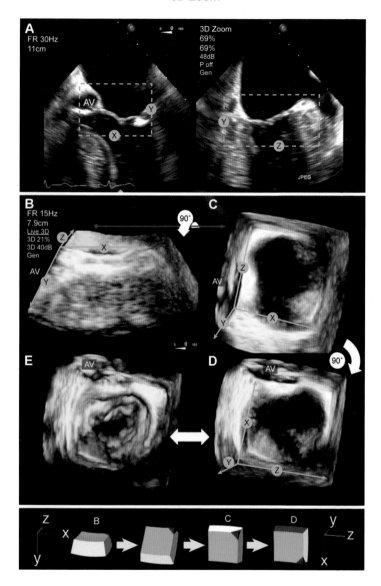

10

Introduction
3D Zoom

3D Zoom mode displays a RT magnified-subsection of 3D volume of varying dimensions with a low FR (< 20 Hz) but good spatial resolution. This RT mode displays a larger sector but unlike the 3D Live mode it requires a couple of extra steps. As an example, 3D Zoom is commonly used to assess the mitral valve (MV).

1. (A) The initial view in 3D Zoom is a biplane preview, shown here are ME 5C and 2C views. Boxes are adjusted for size (X, Y planes), position and elevational width (Z axis) to include the entire MV. The aortic valve (AV) is included in these boxes to help orientate the 3D volume. Probe manipulation or box resizing may be necessary to ensure the boxes encompass the entire MV. Frame rate is lowered with a larger box size and higher line density.

2. (B) Pressing 3D Zoom again generates a pyramid of tissue (3D volume). The dimensions are the size of the original boxes. The face of the volume is the x-y axes. This 3D volume appears in real time so that any probe movement will alter the appearance, but not the size, of the displayed volume.

3. Rotation of the unstored RT 3D volume in space positions it in the appropriate orientation. (C) This dataset is first rotated downward (arrow) so the MV appears en face from the LA side, hidden by over-gain. (D) The en face MV view is now rotated clockwise (arrow) to put the AV at the top of the display.

4. (E) Once positioned the gain is reduced and image optimized to show the MV, here in diastole, in the surgeon's orientation. The 3D volume is now stored.

> NB. 3D Zoom dataset is (mis)labelled as Live 3D on the US machine display.

In the 3D Zoom mode, the entire MV and surrounding structures are shown in clear detail to identify the MV segments and commissures. Spatial resolution is excellent in this mode though the FR (7 Hz) is low. The trade-off here is poor temporal resolution resulting in less smooth playing video clips.

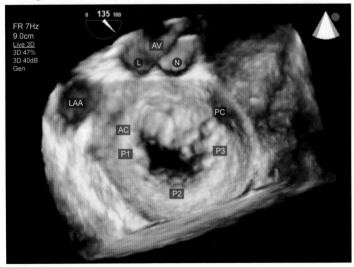

11

Introduction
3D Full Volume

(A) Full Volume (FV) is an ECG gated (4–7 beats) acquisition of a large 3D dataset. It is created from subvolumes stitched together (next page) and synchronized to one cardiac cycle with overlapping ECG traces (arrow). (B–D) FV acquisition begins in a biplane preview, shown are ME AV SAX and LAX views with the same FR 30 Hz. Select the FV acquisition option to optimize (B) volume size (7 beats over large sector), (C) ECG (4 beats over large sector) or (D) frame rate (7 beats over large sector). Low (L) line density expands the sector size at the expense of 3D image resolution. Limited optimization of a 3D FV image necessitates gain (50%) and compression (50%) adjustment in 2D before FV acquisition.

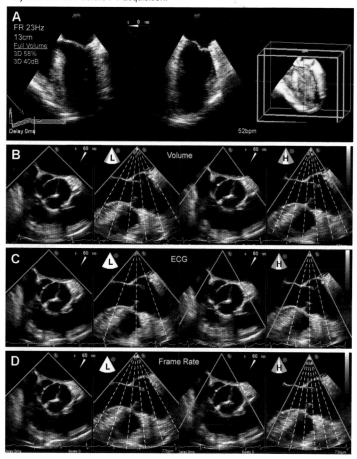

Introduction
3D Full Volume

Once acquired 3D FV images are not shown in RT so the display is unchanged with probe movement. Stored FV 3D datasets can be cropped and orientated into any position. The 20–40 Hz FR (higher 50 Hz with 7 beats) improves temporal resolution. Newer software (ie33, Philips Medical Systems) acquires FV datasets in a different way (see pgs. 14, 15). An irregular heart rhythm, probe or patient movement during FV acquisition creates stitch artifacts which impair image interpretation (see pg. 21).

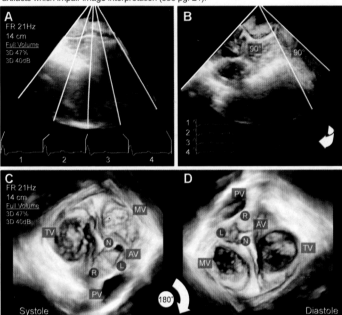

(A) The gated 4 beat FV acquisition of the ME 4C view from the previous page contains 4 subvolumes stitched together. (B) The entire FV is slightly rotated to reveal its pyramidal shape. (C) The base of the heart is obtained by rotating the dataset downwards to view it from the top (atria), shown during systole. (D) The FV dataset can be rotated 180° to orientate it similar to the heart position in the chest, shown during diastole. (E) Compare the 3D images with a pathological specimen.

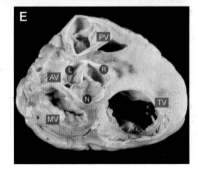

13

Introduction
3D Acquisition

Updated ultrasound machine software (X5-1 for ie33, Philips Medical Systems) using the matrix array probe (X7-2t or X-3, Philips Medical Systems) alters 3D acquisition and displays 3D FV and 3D color Doppler images in RT. In addition 3D volume size and FR can be separately manipulated. For the same-sized 3D voume, the FR can be increased by acquiring the 3D dataset over multiple beats.

The size of the 3D FV acquisition no longer relies on line density or "3D opt" settings (see pg. 12). Instead volume size is now adjustable by independently varying the lateral and elevational widths in RT on the display. The FV is still acquired as subvolumes which now are displayed in RT. Image quality (spatial resolution) in FV acquisition does rely on line density and is optimized by adjusting the RS/speed control.

- RS (resolution) images are acquired with a higher line density (more voxels) and better spatial resolution.
- Speed images have a lower line density (fewer voxels) and a better FR.

Frame rate is now dependent on the number of triggered beats (1, 2, 4, or 6) selected. 3D datasets regardless of size in all 3D modes (Live, Zoom, and FV) can now be acquired and displayed over multiple heartbeats, increasing the FR and temporal resolution. Acquisition time is longer for more beats. The 1 beat acquisition has the lowest FR but is useful because it can be used with arrhythmias as it does not require an ECG.

High volume rate (HVR) acquisition gives the same FR as a 4 subvolume acquisition. The 3D size is the same as 1, 2, 4 subvolumes, only the line density (or voxels) changes. HVR is available in all 3D modes.

Shown on the next page are TTE 3D parasternal LAX images (A, B) Live 3D and (C-E) FV datasets. (A) is a larger 3D Live volume with a 1 beat acquisition and FR (13 Hz); (B) is a smaller 3D volume with a 2 beat acquisition and higher FR (18 Hz). (C) is a FV acquisition over 1 beat (FR 7 Hz) with the adjustable lateral and elevational widths shown. (D) is a smaller 3D FV dataset acquired over 4 beats (FR 44 Hz) that is displayed in RT. (E) is the smaller FV dataset acquired over 1 beat (FR 17 Hz) displayed as a split screen with 2D MPR sectors of the lateral width and elevational width.

Gating	Role	Full Volume	Zoom	Live
	Size[a]	75° × 75°	Variable	60° × 60°
1 beat[b]	Optimize images arrhyth-mias	Displays a 50% cropped RT FV; the size can be adjusted with the eleva-tional and lateral planes. Acquire FV over 1, 2, 4, 6 beats	Displays a biplane preview in which a sector box can be positioned over a ROI. Press 3D Zoom again gives a RT 3D image that can be acquired over 1, 2, or 4 beats.	Displays a live 3D section which can be resized by adjusting the elevational and lateral planes. The RT 3D image can be acquired over 1, 2, or 4 beats.
2 beats				
4 beats	3DQA, stress, Fast HR			
6 beats	Color, contrast		Unavailable	Unavailable

[a] size is lateral x elevational widths
[b] ECG Independent
ROI, region of interest

Introduction
3D Acquisition

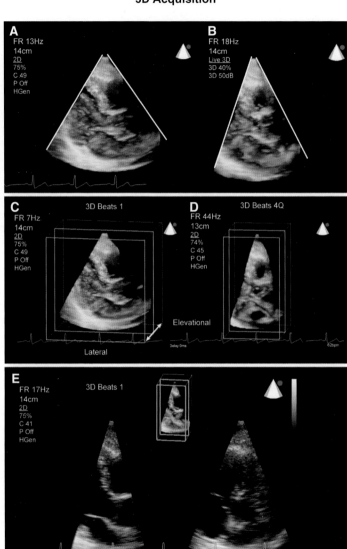

Introduction
3D Color Doppler

Using original machine software (ie33, Philips Medical System) 3D color Doppler requires acquisition of a gated Full Volume dataset. This technology creates only small (up to 60° wide × 60° thick) 3D color Doppler datasets with poor temporal resolution (FR < 10 Hz). The limited sector size may incompletely image color flow in a structure. (A) Color sectors with an appropriate Nyquist limit are centered over the desired area using two orthogonal preview 2D color Doppler views. The largest sector size (green) is obtained by a 10 beat acquisition with low line density. (A) Shown is calcific aortic stenosis in ME AV LAX and SAX views.

Compare TEE color Doppler of an eccentric posterior MR jet that wraps around the LA in (B) 2D and (C) 3D FV rotated to view from LA side. Seven 3D wedge-shaped subvolumes acquired over successive heartbeats are stitched and synchronized to the same cardiac cycle. Stitch artifacts are common. (C) The resulting images appear in a grey scale with superimposed color that gives a crude spatial orientation of the color flow. In 3D color Doppler the broad width of the MR jet is emphasized.

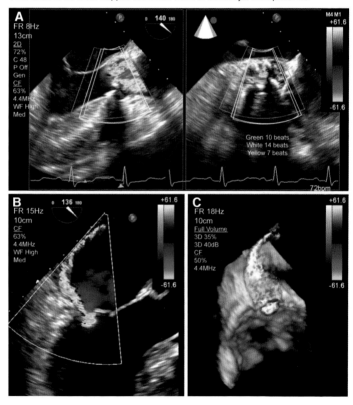

Introduction
3D Color Doppler

Updated machine software (X5-1 for ie33, Philips Medical Systems) allows RT 3D color Doppler images. The sector size is more easily adjustable using elevational and lateral widths to encompass the region of interest. However, the larger the color sector size the lower the FR. This can be partially compensated for by increasing the number of beats acquired (see pg. 14). (A–C) are color Doppler TTE 5C views with normal systolic flow through the aortic valve. (A) 2D view with FR 14 Hz is shown. (B) 3D color Doppler during a 2 beat (FR 5 Hz) acquisition with adjustable lateral and elevational widths is shown. (C) 3D color Doppler 6 beat acquisition which is displayed in RT has a similar FR (14 Hz) to 2D. (D–F) Paravalvular leak around MVR in (D) 2D x Plane color Doppler, RT 3D color Doppler (E) with and (F) without color shows gap (arrow).

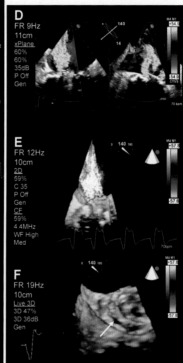

Introduction
3D Image Rotation

A distinct advantage with any 3D image is the opportunity to freely rotate and display it in any orientation. Rotation can be performed either on-line or off-line, on any RT 3D images in the Live and Zoom modes or stored 3D dataset. It is helpful to incorporate an easily identifiable structure (aortic valve, left atrial appendage) to help appropriately orientate the 3D dataset.

While rotation can occur in any plane, for the purposes of this monograph we chose to use the following arrows and terms:

- Axial rotation around the horizontal or vertical axis is indicated by a red arrow. The round tip shows the portion of the 3D image where to position the trackball, the white arrow represents the direction of rotation and the circled number the degrees of rotation. No number represents a variable degree of rotation.
- Z-rotation occurs in the same plane in either clockwise or counterclockwise direction. The circled number is the degrees of rotation.
- Tilt upwards (bottom) or downwards (top) to better expose the corresponding surfaces to view structures.

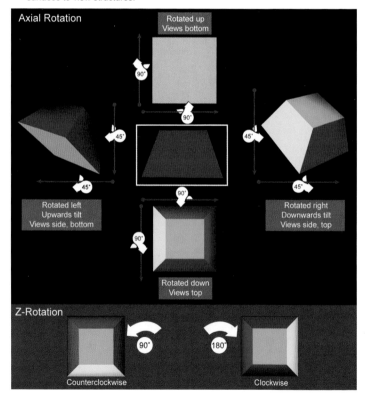

18

Introduction
3D Image Cropping

A stored 3D image can be cropped (or sliced) along three axes (X, Y, Z) using six standard orthogonal planes. A seventh arbitrary cropping plane can be freely manoeuvred in space and aligned to any anatomical structure of interest. Though cropping is performed on-line without using analytical software it cannot be completed in real time as it uses stored 3D images. (A) Shown is the original uncropped 3D FV acquisition of a ME 4C dataset. (B) The crop box removed 50% of the dataset and displayed the interior of the LV. This can be set as an automatic default.

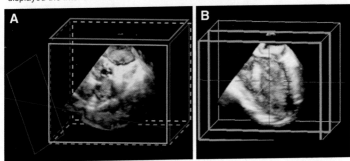

I-crop is a new cropping software (X5-1 on ie33, Philips Medical System) that more easily defines the region of interest (ROI) using multi-planar reconstruction (MPR) in a RT or stored 3D image acquired in any 3D mode. The i-crop preview shows a left MPR pane (red) and right MPR pane (green) and the 3D volume. A crop box in each MPR can be independently sized and positioned over the ROI. As shown here the crop box is positioned parallel to the MV. The cropped 3D volume is displayed in RT in the middle and corresponds to the crop box size and position. The cropped 3D volume can be displayed in six predetermined orientations as indicated by the blue dotted line (**T**op, **Bo**ttom, **R**ight, **L**eft, **F**ront and **Ba**ck) or freely rotated. Shown is the MV from the LA, corresponding to the highlighted top of the crop box.

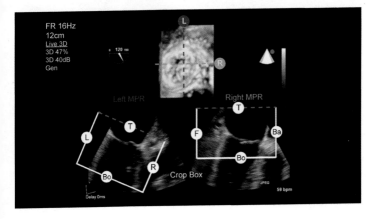

Introduction
3D Image Optimization

Image optimization in 3D begins with adjusting 2D image settings (gain and compression). 3D Live mode is a convenient quick check for 3D image settings with adjustment of gain (A–C shows increasing brown speckles) brightness (D–F shows increasing whiteness) and smoothing (G–I shows a reduction in coarseness of image). These settings can be adjusted in RT or on any stored 3D datasets.

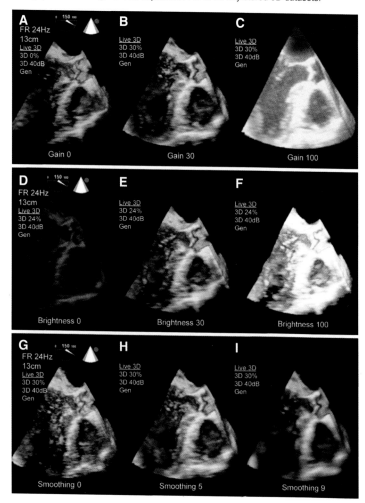

Introduction
3D Artifacts

Dropout is more evident using 3D Live or from reduced gain in all 3D modes. (A) Live 3D ME AV SAX view shows transparent AV cusps during diastole with a visible left coronary artery orifice (arrow), compared to (B) FV of AV from ME AV LAX. Overgain artifacts in 3D imaging appear as brown speckles, shown in 3D Zoom is (C) an obscured MV and (D) a possible mass (arrow) in the LA. (E) Stitch artifacts from an irregular rhythm (arrows) compared with (F) normal 3D FV base of heart views.

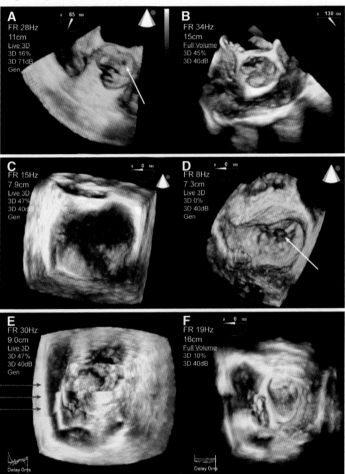

Introduction
Quantification Analysis

(A) 3DQ and (B) 3DQ Advanced are 2 analysis software programs (QLab, Philips Medical Systems) used to optimize and quantify 3D datasets. Availability of this software on the US machine makes off-line exportation of 3D datasets unnecessary. Multiplanar reconstruction (MPRs) of the 3D dataset positions planes through a specific region of interest. Each color coded plane (Green, Red or Blue) can be independently aligned by manipulating a hand cursor. (A) Alignment and measurement of a MR vena contracta area (see pg. 79) and (B) LV function (see pg. 138) are shown.

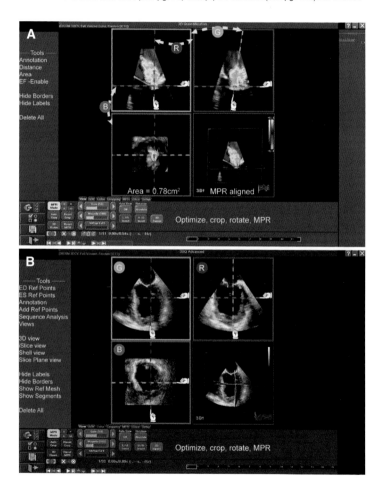

Introduction
Quantification Analysis

Specialized quantification software MVQ (QLab, Philips Medical Systems) for the mitral valve (MV) is available on the ultrasound machine and allows detailed measurements. Analysis of Zoom or Full Volume MV 3D datasets imported into this software generates increasingly detailed basic, standard or advanced models (see pgs. 72, 73). Prompting for the protocol steps (display left) guides the user.

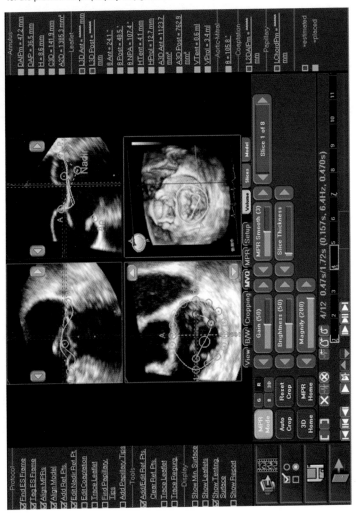

2

3D TEE
Basic Views

A. Vegas et al., *Real-Time Three-Dimensional Transesophageal Echocardiography*, DOI 10.1007/978-1-4614-0665-5_2, © Springer Science+Business Media, LLC 2012

Basic TEE Views
Introduction

The 20 basic TEE views as described by the SCA and ASE are diagrammed here. Conveniently the views are grouped together by the structures being interrogated:

Yellow: Mid-esophageal (ME) views image the LV and MV
Green: ME views image the AV, RVOT, and bicaval
Blue: ME and upper esophageal (UE) views image different regions of the aorta
Orange: Transgastric (TG) views image the LV, RV, and AV for function and spectral Doppler alignment

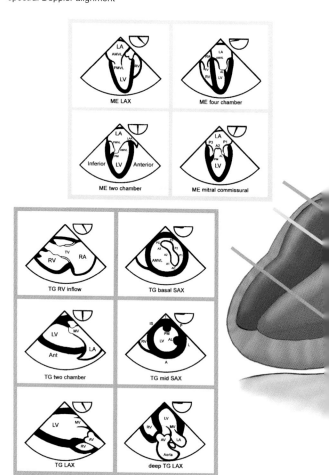

Basic TEE Views
Introduction

Sources
- **Shanewise JS, Cheung AT, Aronson S, et al.** ASE/SCA Guidelines for performing a comprehensive intraoperative multiplane transesophageal echocardiography examination. Anesth Analg 1999; 89:870-84.
- **Flachskampf FA, Decoodt P, Fraser AG, et al.** Guideline from the Working Group: Recommendations for Performing Transesophageal Echocardiography. Eur J Echocardiograph 2001; 2:8-21.

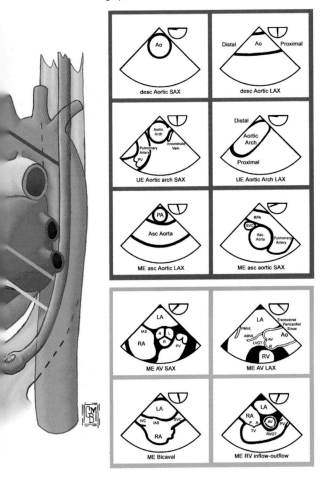

Basic TEE Views
Probe Manipulation

TEE Probe Manipulation
Probe movements (entire probe moves)
1. Advance or withdraw
2. Turn right or left
Knob movements (only probe tip moves)
3. Flex right or left
4. Anteflex or retroflex
Transducer movements (probe stays still)
5. Rotate angle forward
   (0–180°)
6. Rotate angle back (180–0°)

Transducer Planes
- Transverse (0°)
- Longitudinal (90°)
- Omniplane (0–180°)

Image display
- Pie-shaped sector
- Display right (R), left (L)
- Near field (closest to probe)

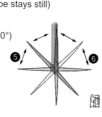

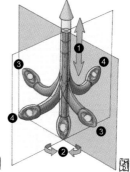

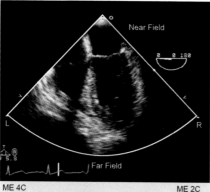

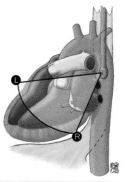

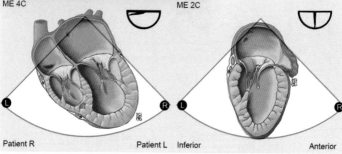

28

Basic TEE Views
TEE Template

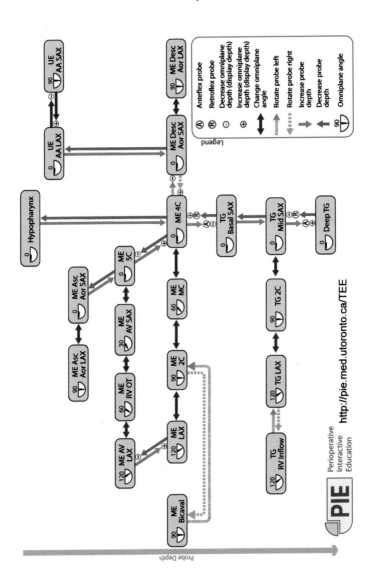

Legend

Ⓐ	Anteflex probe	
Ⓡ	Retroflex probe	
⊖	Decrease omniplane depth (display depth)	
⊕	Increase omniplane depth (display depth)	
↕	Change omniplane angle	
⟹	Rotate probe left	
⟹	Rotate probe right	
→	Increase probe depth	
←	Decrease probe depth	
90	Omniplane angle	

Perioperative
Interactive
Education

PIE

http://pie.med.utoronto.ca/TEE

Probe Depth

Basic TEE Views
ME 4 Chamber

The ME 4C view is obtained by positioning the probe in the mid-esophagus behind the left atrium (LA). The imaging plane is directed through the LA, center of the mitral valve (MV) and left ventricular (LV) apex. A snapshot of the heart shows all four chambers (LA, right atrium RA, LV, right ventricle RV), two valves (MV, tricuspid valve TV), the septa (inter-atrial septum IAS, interventricular septum IVS) and the inferoseptal (IS) and lateral (L) LV walls.

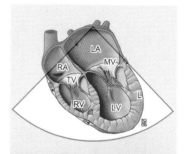

3D Live mode has a reduced sector size that limits imaging of the entire 4C view. Use lateral steer to visualize right and left heart structures (see pg. 9).
3D Full Volume mode (see pg. 135) has a wider sector and is a better choice to image the entire heart.

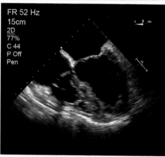

Diagnostic Issues
Chamber enlargement and function
LV systolic function
MV pathology
TV pathology
Atrial septal defect (ASD Primum)
Pericardial effusion

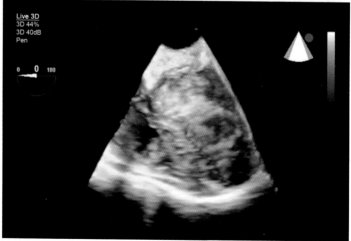

Basic TEE Views
ME Mitral Commissural

In the ME mitral commissural (MC) view, the scanning plane is now orientated at 45°–70° imaging through the left atrium (LA), center of the mitral valve (MV) and left ventricular (LV) apex. The P3 scallop (left), P1 scallop (right) and AMVL (usually A2) is in the middle forming the intermittently seen "trap door." The probe is carefully manipulated to image both the posteromedial (PM) and anterolateral (AL) papillary muscles and LV apex.

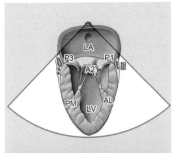

3D Live mode and lateral steer help image the MV, LV walls, and LV apex.
3D Full Volume mode has a wider sector and is a better choice to image the entire heart.

Diagnostic Issues
LA: mass, thrombus
LV systolic function
MV pathology
Coronary sinus flow

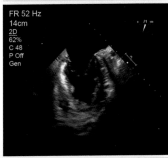

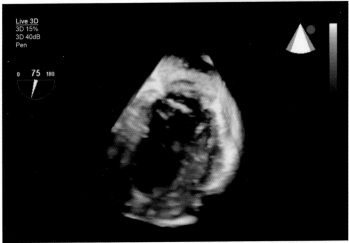

Basic TEE Views
ME 2 Chamber

The ME 2 chamber view is obtained by increasing the omniplane angle to 90° from the ME 4C (0°) or ME mitral commissural (45–60°) views. The right atrium (RA) and right ventricle (RV) are eliminated from the display. This view is orthogonal to the ME 4C view. The image is displayed with the cephalad part (anterior wall) below the left atrial appendage (LAA) to the right and the caudad part (inferior wall) to the left.

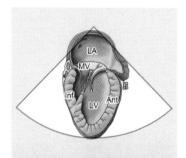

3D Live mode and lateral steer help image the MV, LV walls and LV apex. Tilting the image slightly down allows better visualization of the MV.

3D Full Volume mode has a wider sector and is a better choice to image the entire heart.

Diagnostic Issues
LAA: mass, thrombus
LV systolic function (inferior and anterior)
LV apex pathology
MV pathology
Coronary sinus flow

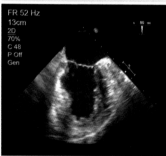

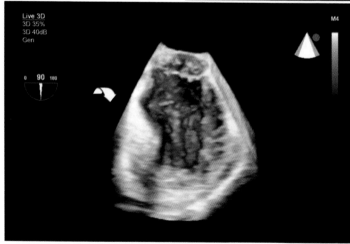

Basic TEE Views
ME LAX

The ME long axis (LAX) view is obtained by increasing the omniplane angle to 120° from the ME 4C (0°) or ME MC (45-60°) or ME 2C (90°) views. The more cephalad structures including the left ventricular outflow tract (LVOT), aortic valve (AV) and the proximal ascending aorta are lined up on the display right. The apex of the left ventricle (LV) and inferolateral (IL) and anteroseptal (AS) walls are seen.

3D Live mode and lateral steer help image the MV, AV, LV walls and LV apex.
3D Full Volume mode has a wider sector and is a better choice to image the aortic root and entire LV.

Diagnostic Issues
MV pathology
LV systolic function
IVS pathology (VSD)
LVOT pathology
AV pathology
Aortic root pathology

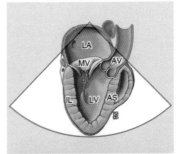

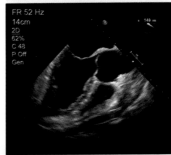

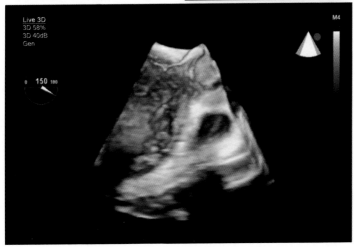

Basic TEE Views
ME AV LAX

The ME aortic valve (AV) LAX view is obtained by decreasing the display depth from the ME LAX view (120°). The left ventricular outflow tract (LVOT), AV and the proximal ascending aorta are lined up on the display right and the remainder of the mitral valve (MV) and left ventricle (LV) are eliminated from the image.

3D Live mode and lateral steer help center the AV in the image display. Rotating the image 90° (arrows) allows visualization from either the LVOT or aorta. The limited sector size shows only half of these perspectives.

3D Full Volume (see pg. 85) or **3D Zoom modes** have a wider sector and are better choices to image the aortic root or LVOT.

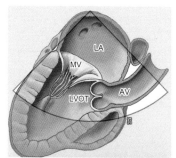

Diagnostic Issues
AV pathology
Aortic root dimensions
Aortic root pathology
LVOT pathology
MV anterior leaflet
Ventricular septal defect (VSD)

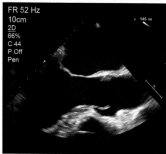

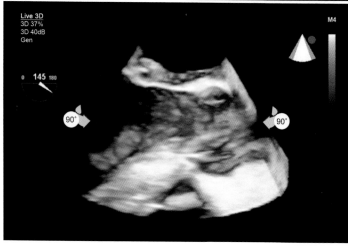

34

Basic TEE Views
ME AV SAX

From the ME 4C view, the probe is withdrawn until the aortic valve (AV) is positioned centrally. To obtain the ME AV SAX view, increase the omniplane angle to 30°–45° with slight anteflexion to align the imaging plane parallel to the AV annulus. All three aortic cusps appear symmetrical. Withdraw the probe to image the orifices of the left main and right coronary arteries.

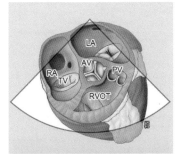

3D Live mode is suboptimal to image the thin AV cusps as significant dropout is present unless the gain is increased.

3D Full Volume (see pg. 84) or **3D Zoom modes** improve cusp definition and visualization of the coronary artery orifices. Rotating the image 180° (arrow) shows the AV from the LVOT.

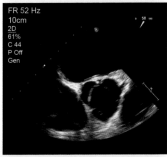

Diagnostic Issues

AV morphology
AV planimetry
AI location
ASD secundum
LA size (anterior–posterior diameter)

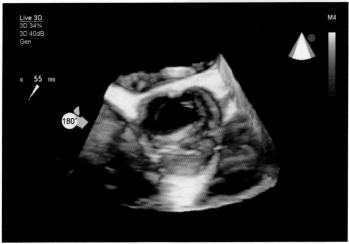

Basic TEE Views
ME RV Inflow–Outflow

Aptly named, this view images the right ventricular (RV) inflow from the tricuspid valve (TV) on the display left and RV outflow tract (RVOT) through the pulmonic valve (PV) on the display right in a single view. This view is obtained from the ME AV SAX view (30°) by increasing the omniplane angle to 60–75°. An off axis image of the aortic valve (AV) is displayed centrally.

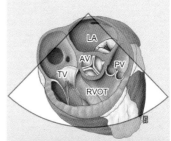

3D Live mode narrow sector only images the RVOT. Lateral steer (arrows, see pg. 9) helps to better image the TV to the left and PV to the right.
3D Full Volume (see pg. 12) or **3D Zoom modes** have a wider sector and are better choices to image the entire RVOT.

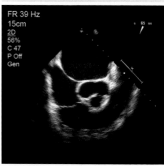

Diagnostic Issues
Pulmonic valve pathology
Pulmonary artery pathology
RVOT pathology
TV pathology
TV Doppler
Atrial septal defect (ASD secundum)
Ventricular septal defect (VSD)

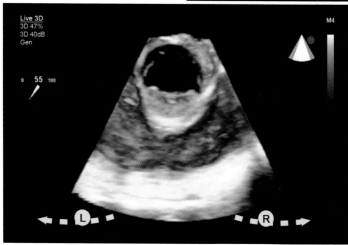

Basic TEE Views
ME Bicaval

The view is obtained from the ME 2C view (90°) by turning the entire probe to the patient's right towards the superior vena cava (SVC) and inferior vena cava (IVC). The transducer plane cuts through the left atrium (LA), right atrium (RA), and LAX of the IVC and SVC. The structures are displayed with the LA at the sector apex (closest to probe), RA in the far field and caudad IVC (left) and cephalad SVC (right).

3D Live mode narrow sector images the inter-atrial septum (IAS) through the LA. Lateral steer helps to better image the SVC (right) and IVC (left). Tilting the image down slightly shows the IAS from the LA perspective. A catheter is seen in the SVC.
3D Full Volume (see pgs. 204, 205) or **3D Zoom modes** have a wider sector and are better choices to image the entire IAS.

Diagnostic Issues
IAS: Atrial septal defect (ASD)
Mass
SVC/IVC flow
Venous catheters
Pacemaker wires
Venous cannula position (SVC/IVC)

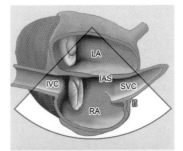

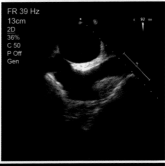

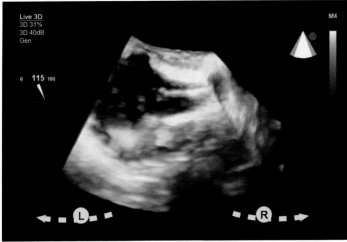

Basic TEE Views
TG Basal SAX

The TG basal SAX view is obtained by withdrawing the probe from the TG mid-papillary SAX view or as the probe is advanced into the stomach at 0°. This permits a TG view of the mitral valve (MV) that is parallel to the MV annulus with the posterior mitral valve leaflet (PMVL) on the display right and the anterior mitral valve leaflet (AMVL) to the left. The posterior commissure (PC) is closest to the probe as are P3 and A3; the anterior commissure (AC) is in the far field.

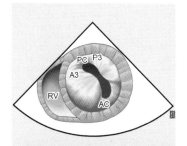

3D Live mode the narrow sector poorly images the thin MV leaflets and provides little additional information. The left ventricular (LV) walls are also incompletely imaged. **3D Full Volume or 3D Zoom modes** are not often used to image the MV from this view as ME views provide better MV 3D images.

Diagnostic Issues
MV: pathology, origin MR
LV: basal segment function
Ventricular septal defect (VSD)

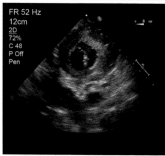

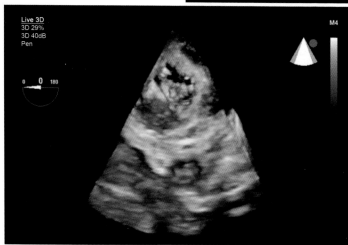

38

Basic TEE Views
TG mid SAX

The TG views are obtained by advancing the probe in a neutral position into the stomach and applying varying degrees of anteflexion. In the TG mid-papillary SAX view (0°), the left ventricle (LV) is imaged in SAX with 6 LV segments (ASE/SCA 17 segment model; see pg. 140) viewed at once. Manipulate the probe to center the LV cavity and slightly increase the transducer angle to obtain a symmetrical circular LV.

3D Live mode the narrow sector cannot image all the LV walls simultaneously.
3D Full Volume from the ME views is the preferred method to assess LV function (see pgs. 138, 139).

Diagnostic Issues
LV cavity size
LV wall thickness
LV systolic function
Hemodynamic instability
IVS motion
Ventricular septal defect (VSD)

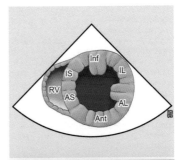

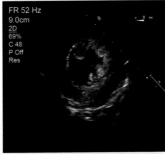

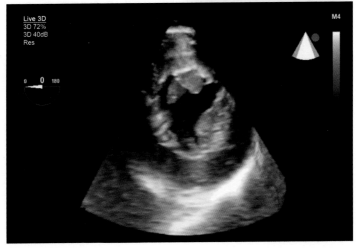

Basic TEE Views
TG 2 Chamber

The TG 2C view is obtained from the TG mid-papillary SAX view (0°) by increasing the transducer angle to 75°–90°. This images the left ventricle (LV) in LAX and the subvalvular structures of the mitral valve (MV). This view is similar to the ME 2C view now turned 90° with the probe closest to the inferior (Inf) wall of the LV (apex of sector).

3D Live mode images the LV walls, papillary muscles and MV. The narrow sector cuts off the MV and may require lateral steer.

3D Full Volume mode has a wider sector but is not often used in this view.

Diagnostic Issues
LV systolic function
MV subvalvular apparatus
MV pathology

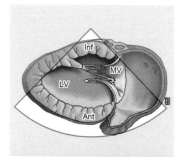

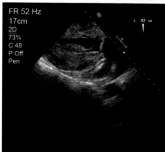

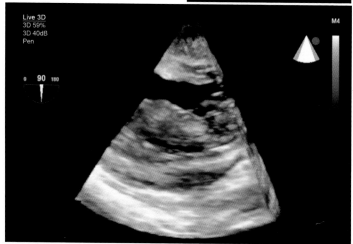

Basic TEE Views
TG LAX

The TG LAX view is developed from the TG 2C view (90°) by increasing the transducer angle to 120°. The left ventricular outflow tract (LVOT) and aortic valve (AV) appear on the display right, depending on the depth settings. This view is similar to the ME AV LAX view and permits better Doppler alignment of the LVOT and AV. The mitral valve and subvalvular structures are also seen.

3D Live mode the narrow sector and thin AV cusps result in poor imaging of the AV. Lateral steer and increasing gain may improve imaging of the AV.
3D Full Volume color mode may be used to assess flow through the AV.

Diagnostic Issues
MV: leaflets, subvalvular
LV systolic function
AV Doppler gradient
LVOT Doppler gradient
Ventricular septal defect (VSD)
Prosthetic AV function

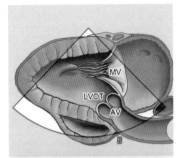

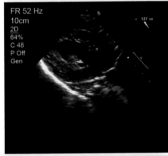

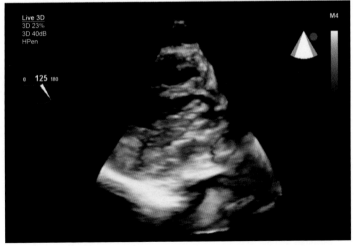

41

Basic TEE Views
TG Deep LAX

To obtain the deep TG LAX view (0°), the probe is advanced deep into the stomach and anteflexed. Leftward flexion may be necessary to place the left ventricular outflow tract (LVOT) and aortic valve (AV) in the center of the screen. This image may be utilized in measuring the Doppler velocity of flow across the LVOT and the AV.

3D Live mode the narrow sector, thin AV cusps and far field position result in poor imaging of the AV.
3D Full Volume color mode may be used to assess flow through the AV.

Diagnostic Issues
AV pathology
AV spectral Doppler
Prosthetic AV function
LVOT spectral Doppler
LVOT pathology
Ventricular septal defect (VSD)

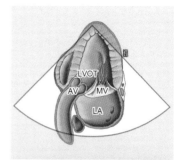

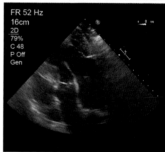

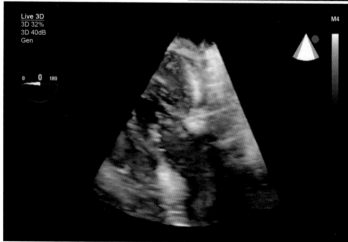

Basic TEE Views
TG RV Inflow

The TG RV inflow view (120°) reveals a long axis view of the right ventricle (RV), with the apex of the RV to the left and the anterior (Ant) free wall in the far field. It is obtained from the TG basal SAX view (0°), by turning the probe to the right to center the tricuspid valve (TV) and increasing the omniplane angle to 120°. The subvalvular structures of the TV are well seen.

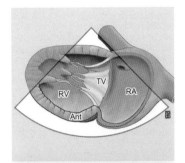

3D Live mode the narrow sector and thin TV cusps result in poor imaging of the RV and TV. Lateral steer to the left may image more of the RV.
3D Full Volume mode has a wider sector but is not often used in this view.

Diagnostic Issues
TV pathology
RV systolic function
Right atrial (RA) mass

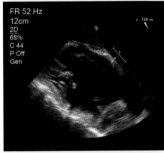

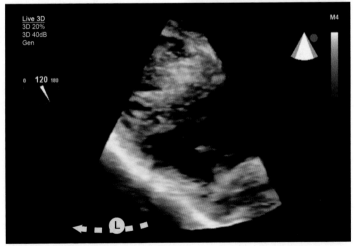

43

Basic TEE Views
ME Descending Aorta SAX

The descending thoracic aorta is visualized in SAX (0°) by turning the probe to the left from the ME 4C view (0°). The near field image of the circular aorta represents the right anterior wall of the aorta. Advance and withdraw the probe to image the entire descending aorta. Decrease the display depth.

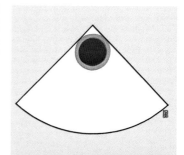

3D Live mode with a slight tilt down better images a SAX section of the aorta intimal surface. The near field aortic wall is, however, poorly visualized.

3D Full Volume mode (see pg. 175) is a better choice to image a wider sector of the aorta and the thin wall of a dissection flap (see pg. 179).

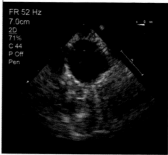

Diagnostic Issues
Aorta atherosclerosis
Aorta dissection
Aorta aneurysm
Left pleural effusion
AI severity PW Doppler
IABP position

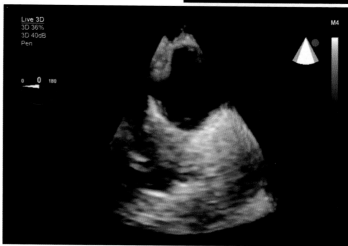

44

Basic TEE Views
ME Descending Aorta LAX

From the descending thoracic aorta SAX view (0°) the transducer angle is increased to 90° to obtain the descending aortic LAX view. The distal aorta is to the display left and the proximal aorta to the display right.

3D Live mode with a slight tilt down better images a section of the aorta intimal surface. The near field aortic wall is, however, poorly visualized.
3D Full Volume mode (see pg. 173) is a better choice to image a wider sector of the aorta and the thin wall of a dissection flap (see pg. 179).

Diagnostic Issues
Aorta atherosclerosis
Aorta dissection
Aorta aneurysm
AI severity PW Doppler
IABP position

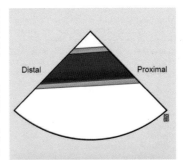

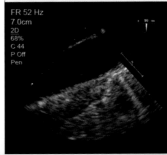

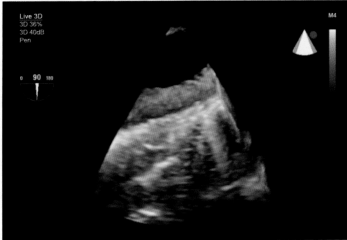

Basic TEE Views
UE Aortic Arch LAX

From the descending thoracic aorta SAX view (0°), the probe is withdrawn cephalad to the upper esophagus (UE). The circular shape of the descending thoracic aorta changes to an oblong shape of the transverse aortic arch (0°). The proximal aortic arch is to the display left and the distal arch to the right. Further probe withdrawal may image the great vessels of the head and neck.

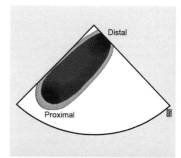

3D Live mode with a slight tilt better images a section of the aorta intimal surface. The near field aortic wall is, however, poorly visualized.
3D Full Volume mode (see pg. 173) is a better choice to image a wider sector of the aorta and aortic pathology.

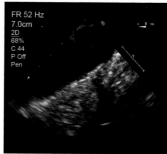

Diagnostic Issues
Aorta atherosclerosis
Aorta dissection
Aorta aneurysm
AI severity PW Doppler

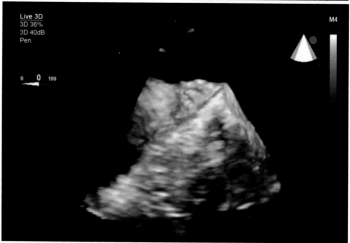

Basic TEE Views
UE Aortic Arch SAX

From the upper esophageal (UE) aortic arch LAX view (0°), increasing the transducer angle to 60–90° obtains the UE aortic arch SAX view. With probe manipulation the proximal origin of the left subclavian artery and innominate vein is seen in the upper right display. The pulmonic valve (PV) and main pulmonary artery (PA) in LAX are seen in the lower left display.

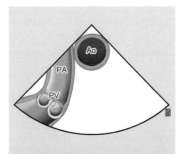

3D Live mode with a slight tilt down better images a narrow section of the PA intimal surface. The thin PV cusps are poorly seen.

3D Full Volume mode is a better choice to image a wider sector of the aorta and the thin PV cusps (see pg. 110).

Diagnostic Issues
Aorta atherosclerosis
Aorta dissection
Aorta aneurysm
Pulmonic valve pathology
Patent ductus arteriosus (PDA)
Swan–Ganz catheter position

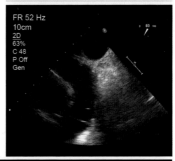

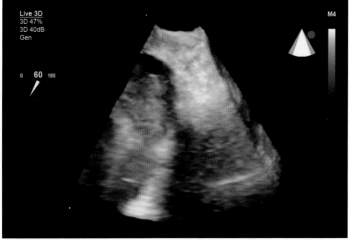

Basic TEE Views
ME Ascending Aorta SAX

The ME ascending aorta SAX view (0–10°) is obtained by withdrawing the probe from the ME aortic valve SAX view (30°) and rotating the omniplane angle back to 0°. This view is also obtained from the mid-ascending aorta LAX (120°) by decreasing the omniplane angle to 0–10° to image superior vena cava (SVC) in SAX, ascending aorta (Asc. Aorta) in SAX and the right pulmonary artery (RPA) in LAX.

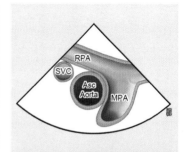

3D Live, Zoom, Full Volume modes even with a slight tilt down provide little additional information in 3D for this view.

Diagnostic Issues
Aorta atherosclerosis
Aorta dissection
Aorta aneurysm
Pulmonary embolism
Swan–Ganz catheter position

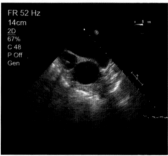

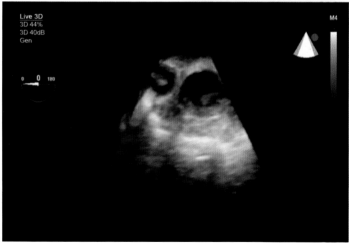

48

Basic TEE Views
ME Ascending Aorta LAX

The mid-ascending aorta (Asc. Aorta) in LAX may be visualized from the ME AV LAX (120°), by withdrawing the probe to image the right pulmonary artery (RPA) in SAX.

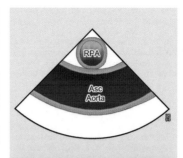

3D Live mode with a slight tilt down images a section of the aorta intimal surface. The image quality is frequently poor as this is a difficult 2D image to obtain.

3D Full Volume or Zoom modes may provide better images for the ascending aorta in LAX.

Diagnostic Issues
Aorta atherosclerosis
Aorta dissection
Aorta aneurysm
AI flow
Aortic stenosis flow
Swan–Ganz catheter in RPA
Pericardial effusion in transverse sinus

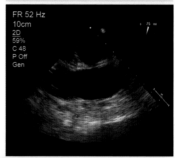

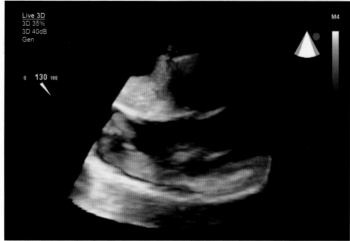

49

Basic TEE Views
ME Left Atrial Appendage

The left atrial appendage (LAA) view is obtained by reducing the image depth from the ME RVOT view and adjusting the omniplane angle between 60° and 80°. The LAA is seen above the mitral valve (MV) and aortic valve (AV). The left upper pulmonary vein (LUPV) is above, more posterior and closer to the probe.

3D Live mode shows only half of the LAA.
3D Full Volume and Zoom modes image the entire LAA. The orifice of the LAA can be seen from a rotated surgical orientation (see pg. 219).

Diagnostic Issues
LAA pathology
LUPV flow

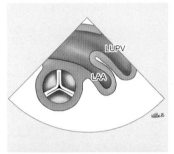

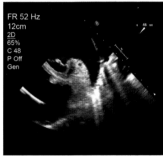

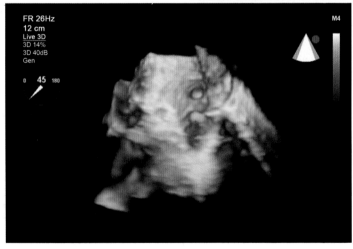

Basic TEE Views
TG Inferior Vena Cava

The transgastric (TG) inferior vena cava (IVC) LAX view is obtained by advancing the probe to image the TG mid-SAX view (0°). Turn the probe right to find the liver, withdraw to find the IVC as it enters the right atrium (RA). Adjust the probe and omniplane angle to identify the hepatic vein (HV) as it enters the IVC.

3D Live mode images the hepatic vein well. The lumen of the IVC is difficult to visualize due to dropout of the wall closest to the probe.

Diagnostic Issues
Tricuspid regurgitation
Mass (tumor, thrombus)
IVC cannula position
IVC respiratory variation

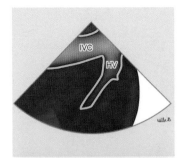

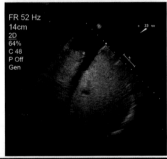

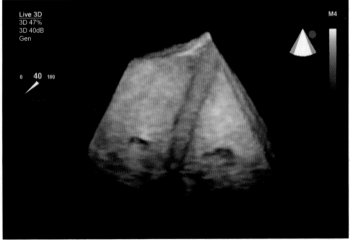

3

Native Cardiac Valves

A. Vegas et al., *Real-Time Three-Dimensional Transesophageal Echocardiography*, DOI 10.1007/978-1-4614-0665-5_3, © Springer Science+Business Media, LLC 2012

Mitral Valve
Normal Anatomy

Fibrous Skeleton (3 parts)
1. Base of aortic valve (AV)
2. Right + left fibrous trigones
   intertrigonal distance (ITD)
   between R and L trigones
   ITD = AV diameter/0.8
3. Smaller fibrous area between
   RCC and pulmonary artery

"Aortic curtain" is fibrous and common
to aortic + mitral valves

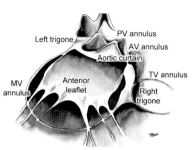

Mitral Annulus
- Posterior annulus has little fibrous tissue
  which predisposes to P2 prolapse
- Saddle-shaped (hyperbolic paraboloid)
  highest ME AV LAX view (120°)
- Changes shape
  circle (diastole): 40% larger
  "D" shape (systole): smaller
- Measure annulus in diastole: use 2
  views (0°/90°), normal size (29 ± 4 mm)
- Flexible annuloplasty ring accommodates
  shape change

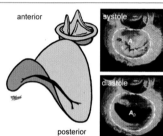

Mitral Valve Leaflets (4 anatomic leaflets)

1. Anterior (AMVL): 2/3 MV area, 1/3 MV annulus
2. Posterior (PMVL): 2/3 MV annulus, 3 scallops
3. Anterior commissure (AC)
4. Posterior commissure (PC)
Leaflet nomenclature (next page)
Leaflet thickness ≤ 4 mm

MV leaflet surface area twice the annulus area (4–6 cm²) so
creates a large leaflet coaptation area (30%).

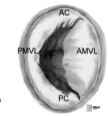

Chordae Tendineae (3 orders)
1st: leaflet free margin
2nd: ventricular leaflet aspect
3rd: ventricle wall to PMVL only
stay chordae: attach to AMVL important
  for MV geometry
Papillary Muscles (PM)
Anterolateral: A2, A1, Ac, P1, P2
Posteromedial: A2, A3, Pc, P3, P2
Posterior PM has single artery supply
(RCA or obtuse marginal of circumflex)
so is prone to ischemia.

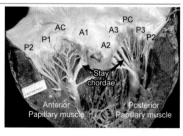

Mitral Valve Nomenclature

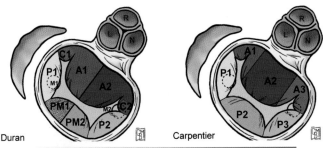

Duran   Carpentier

Leaflet Nomenclature		
Anatomic	**Duran**	**Carpentier**
Posterior leaflet (scallops)		
Lateral	P1	P1
Middle	PM (1/2)	P2
Medial	P2	P3
Commissural leaflets		
Anterolateral	C1	Ac com
Posteromedial	C2	Pc com
Anterior leaflet (segments)		
	A1	A1
	A2	A2
		A3

Carpentier classification of dysfunction is based on the systolic position of the mitral leaflets in relation to the annular plane. Carpentier's pathophysiologic triad to describe mitral regurgitation (MR) consists of the disease, lesions and dysfunction.

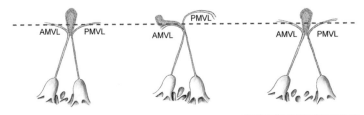

Type 1	**Type 2**	**Type 3**
Normal leaflet motion, central MR typically from annular dilatation or leaflet perforation	Excessive leaflet motion, leaflet tip above the annular plane, resulting in eccentric MR (opposite to prolapsed segment)	Restricted leaflet motion, 3a: both systole and diastole as in subvalvular fibrosis 3b: only systole as in ventricular remodeling

Mitral Valve
2D Assessment

TEE for the Mitral Valve Apparatus

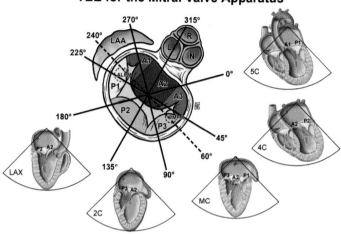

Surgeon's View of the Mitral Valve Apparatus

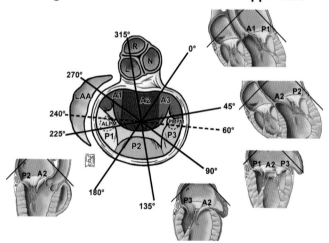

Mitral Valve
2D Assessment

xPlane: The MV is imaged through the entire 360° with xPlane showing scallops as diagrammed on the previous page. The reference image is on the display left, with an orthogonal view on the right. The probe is held stationary.

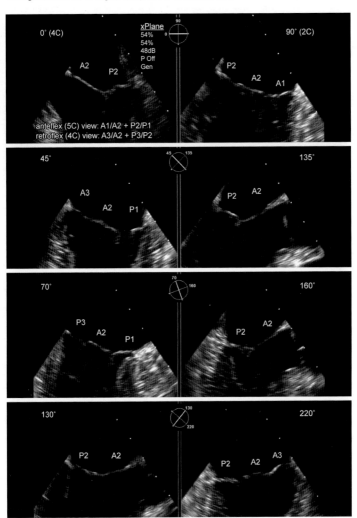

Mitral Valve
3D Live and Zoom

The MV is incompletely imaged using **3D Live**. Various 3D Live ME views can be acquired and tilted downward to assess different portions of the MV. (A) 3D Live ME 4C view tilted slightly downward to view the posterior commissure (PC), the leaflet edges are labeled as A2 and P2. (B) 3D Live ME AV LAX view rotated downward views the anterior commissure (AC); the anterior leaflet is adjacent to the aortic valve (AV).

(C) The MV is imaged using TEE **3D Zoom** and rotated to display it in the surgeon's orientation as seen from the LA (see pgs. 10,11). In this image the scallops of the posterior mitral valve leaflet (PMVL) are apparent. Note the AV (**N**on and **L**eft cusps) is displayed at the top of the image and the left atrial appendage (LAA) to the left. (D) Compare with a view at the time of surgery.

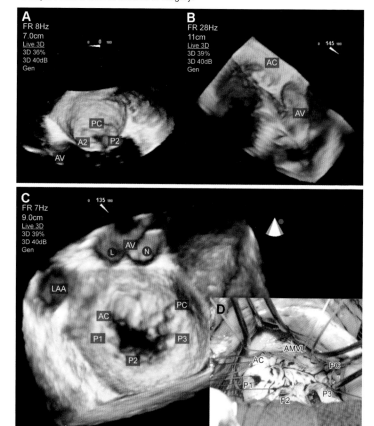

Mitral Valve
3D Full Volume

Systematic use of additional perspectives ('angled views') reveals important details of both commissures and the adjacent leaflet segments. These views enable accurate RT definition of the involved segments in MV prolapse (MVP) and is less time consuming than off-line postprocessing. (A) **Anterolateral (AL) view:** 90–110° anticlockwise rotation, 60–70° backward tilt of en face view (C, pg. 58). Best to evaluate involvement of the anterolateral commissure, A1 and P1. (B) **Scallop view:** 70–90° anticlockwise rotation and 20–30° medial tilt of the AL view, best shows the 3 posterior leaflet scallops. (C) **Posteromedial (PM) view:** 90° anticlockwise rotation and slight forward tilt of AL view. Best to assess the posteromedial commissure, P3 and A3. Shown are 3D Full Volume ME MV images of flail P2 (arrow).

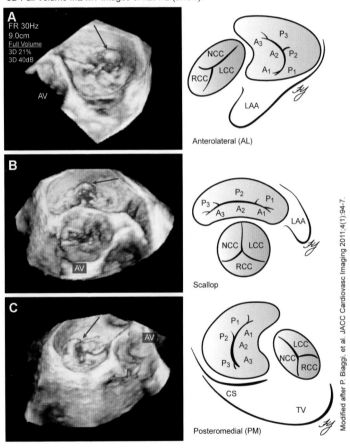

Anterolateral (AL)

Scallop

Posteromedial (PM)

Modified after P. Biaggi. et al. JACC Cardiovasc Imaging 2011;4(1):94-7.

Mitral Valve
Mitral Regurgitation

1. Etiology of regurgitation: (normal finding in 40% of patients)
   - Leaflet: prolapse, flail, myxomatous, rheumatic, endocarditis
   - Annulus: dilated (LV/LA), mitral annular calcification (MAC)
   - Chordae: rupture, elongation, shortening, tenting, SAM
   - Papillary muscle rupture, LV dysfunction
2. 2D/3D findings:
   - Leaflets: thickened (> 5 mm), calcific, malcoaptation, prolapse, flail, vegetation
   - Annulus: MAC, size (mid-diastole 29 ± 4 mm)
3. Doppler findings:
   - Color: turbulent systolic flow from LV to LA, flow acceleration below MV
   - Color: jet direction: central, posterior, anterior
   - Color: area mapping (trace mosaic area), vena contracta (narrowest width), proximal flow convergence (PISA)
   - CW: systolic flow above baseline, velocity 5–6 m/s, density $\propto$ MR, contour parabolic or early peaking, triangular shape in severe MR
   - PW: mitral inflow velocity > 1.5 m/s with moderate–severe MR (no MS), A-wave predominance excludes severe MR
   - PW: pulmonary veins systolic flow reversal specific but not sensitive, absent if large LA. Eccentric jet look in contralateral pulmonary vein.
4. LA enlarged (> 55 mm AP diameter), LA:RA ratio > 1
5. LV dimensions and systolic function are important prognostic factors and indicators for surgery. Dilated due to volume overload.
   - LV size: ESD > 55 mm
   - Systolic function: initially good, but worsens
6. Regurgitation severity (severe) based on the following (ASE):
   - Specific:
     - Vena contracta: > 7 mm with central jet (> 40% LA) or any eccentric jet
     - Flow convergence (PISA): > 9 mm (Nyquist 40 cm/s) central jet
     - Pulmonary vein systolic flow reversal
   - Supportive:
     - CW Doppler dense, triangular, E-wave dominant MV inflow (> 1.2 m/s)
     - Enlarged LV and LA size
   - Quantitative:
     - Regurgitant volume (RegV): > 60 cc
     - Regurgitant fraction (RF): > 50%
     - Effective regurgitant orifice area (EROA): > 0.4 cm^2

What to tell the surgeon:
Pre CPB
- Myxomatous, calcified, prolapsed/flail segments, annular size, MAC
- Direction and severity of MR jets, pulmonary vein flow (blunted/reversed)
- LV size and function
Post CPB
- Post-repair mitral leaflet morphology, prosthetic valve function
- Residual MR, impaired mitral inflow (? stenotic)
- Complications repair: SAM, posterior wall (circumflex art), atrioventricular groove separation, AV non-coronary cusp trauma
- LV / RV function, severity TR

Mitral Valve
Mitral Regurgitation

Mitral Regurgitation Severity Assessment (AHA/ASE)

Method	Mild	Moderate	Severe
CW Doppler signal strength	faint	mod	dense
Jet area mapping (cm²)[b]	< 4	4–10	> 10
Jet area (JA) / Left atrial (LA) area (%)	< 20	20–40	> 40
Pulmonary venous doppler (S wave)	normal	blunt	reverse
Regurgitant volume (cc)	< 30	30–59	≥ 60
Regurgitant fraction (%)	< 30	30–49	≥ 50
Vena contracta (mm)[b]	< 3	4–6	≥ 7
Effective regurgitant orifice area (cm²)	< 0.20	0.20–0.39	≥ 0.4
PISA radius (mm)[a]	< 4	4–9	> 10

Assess regurgitation severity under physiologic conditions (SBP, afterload and LV function).
Use appropriate Nyquist velocity [a]40 cm/s, [b]50–60 cm/s and color gain.
Adapted from Zoghbi W, et al. J Am Soc Echocardiogr 2003;16:777-802

Jet Area Mapping
- Trace mosaic jet area
- Nyquist 50–60 cm/s
- Physiology dependent
- Underestimates if eccentric jets
- Useful if multiple jets

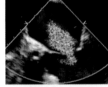 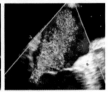

Moderate 4-10 cm²   Severe > 10 cm²

Vena Contracta
- Narrowest diameter, measure above flow acceleration region
- Nyquist 50–60 cm/s
- Useful if eccentric jets
- Not used if multiple jets
- Best measured in ME AV LAX view

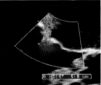 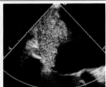

Moderate 4-6 mm   Severe > 7 mm

PISA (EROA)
- Radius proximal flow convergence
- Nyquist 40 cm/s
- Less useful if eccentric
- Not used if multiple jets

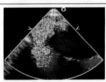 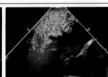

Moderate 4-10 mm   Severe > 10 mm

CW Doppler
- Density, compare with forward flow
- Contour (complete)

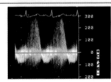 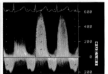

Mitral Valve
Barlow's Disease

Barlow's disease is a degenerative disease of the MV from myxoid infiltration resulting in excessive leaflet tissue. An example is shown from the LA side (A) using 3D Zoom, (B) at surgery and in the (C) 2D TEE ME Mitral Commissural view with bileaflet prolapse and severe central MR. The MV annulus is often displaced into the LA complicating the repair. (D) A 3D model reconstruction shows bileaflet prolapse.

Source: Eriksson M, et al. J Am Soc Echocardiogr 2005; 18:1014-22.

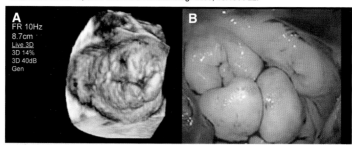

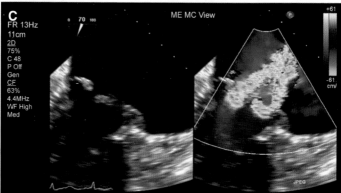

Barlow's Mitral Valve

- Excessively thick leaflets
- Prolapse both leaflets
- Central or eccentric MR
- Annular dilatation
- Annulus displacement into LA
- Chordal elongation and thickened
- Chordal rupture uncommon
- Complex repair

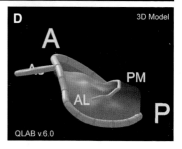

Mitral Valve
Fibroelastic Disease

Fibroelastic degeneration of the MV in two patients with an isolated P2 prolapse with flail tip (P2) and torn chordae (arrow). (A, B) Examples are shown from the LA side in the surgeon's orientation using RT TEE 3D Zoom. (C) Compare 2D ME 4C view of the MV with color Doppler showing severe anterior directed MR. (D) Reconstructed 3D model shows prolapsed segment.

Source: O'Gara P, et al. JACC Cardiol Img 2008; 1:221-37.

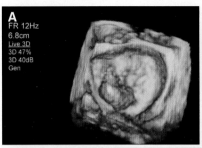
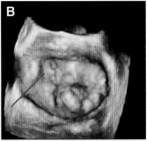

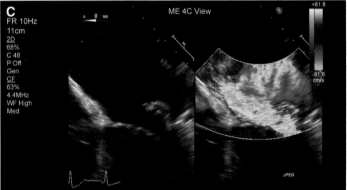

Fibroelastic Disease

- Normal leaflet thickness
- Isolated segment prolapse
- Eccentric MR
- ± Annular dilatation
- No annulus displacement
- Chordal rupture
- Simple repair

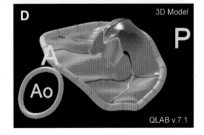

Mitral Valve
A1 Prolapse

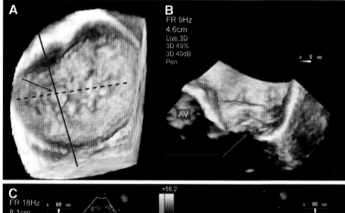

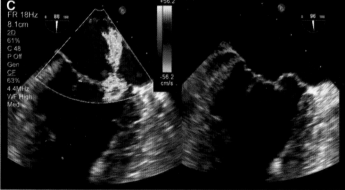

Patient with isolated A1 prolapse from fibroelastic degeneration of the MV. (A) TEE 3D Zoom of A1 prolapse (arrow) is shown from the LA side in the surgeon's orientation. (B) A sagittal section through the prolapsed A1 segment, Fig. A solid line, is cropped and rotated. Compare dotted line Fig. A with (C) 2D TEE ME 2C view and color Doppler which best shows the prolapse and MR. (D) Reconstructed 3D model shows prolapsed A1 (in red) at the anterior commissure.

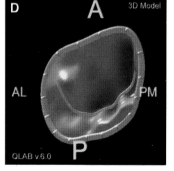

Source: Grewal J, et al. J Am Soc Echocardiogr 2009; 22:34-41.

Mitral Valve
Mitral Annular Calcification

Patients with restricted MV leaflet motion from calcification are shown. One patient has an isolated block of calcium (arrow) in the P2 segment of the MV. This is shown in (A) 3D Zoom from the LA side in the surgeon's orientation compared with a (B) 2D TEE ME view. Another patient has severe annular calcification in the setting of aortic stenosis shown using (C) 3D Zoom and (D) 2D ME color Doppler views. (E) Reconstructed 3D model shows restriction of the posterior mitral valve leaflet.

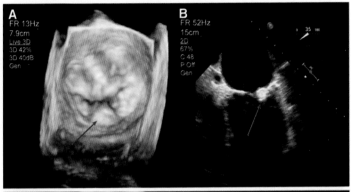

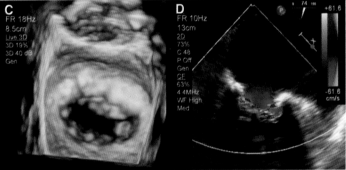

Restricted Mitral Valve

- Thick leaflets, calcium
- No prolapse
- Restricted mobility (open, close)
- Annular calcium
- Chordal restriction
- Difficult repair, valve replacement

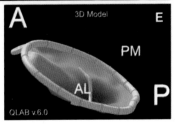

Mitral Valve
Mitral Stenosis

1. Etiology of stenosis:
   - Valvular: rheumatic, calcific (MAC), carcinoid, SLE, congenital, drugs
   - Subvalvular: mass, myxoma
2. 2D/3D findings:
   - Annulus: Ca^{2+}, size (end diastole)
   - Leaflets: Ca^{2+}, thickness (> 4 mm), mobility, diastolic doming "hockey stick"
   - Chordae: Ca^{2+}, thickened, extent of subvalvular involvement
   - Planimeter MVA in TG basal SAX view or 3D off-line
3. Doppler findings:
   - Color: turbulent diastolic flow, proximal flow acceleration
   - PW/CW: peak velocity > 3 m/s, peak/mean P gradient
     - Note elevated transmitral inflow also occurs with high cardiac output, MR and restrictive diastolic filling
   - Pressure half-time (PHT) for native mitral valve area (MVA)
4. Stenosis severity (severe):
   - Peak velocity > 3 m/s
   - Mean pressure gradient > 10 mmHg
   - Mitral valve area < 1.0 cm^2 (planimetry, PHT)
5. Coexisting MR (overestimates measured pressure gradients)
6. LA enlargement (LAX view: A-P diameter > 45 mm), smoke, thrombus in LAA
7. PASP (estimate from TR jet)
8. Coexisting TR severity
9. RV function: dilated, hypertrophy, IVS paradoxical motion
10. LV function: small underfilled, SWMA (postero-basal segment)

Severity Assessment (EAE/ASE Guidelines)

	Valve Area (cm^2)	Mean Gradient (mmHg)	PHT (ms)	Peak Pulmonary artery P (mmHg)
Normal	4–6		40–70	20–30
Mild	> 1.5	< 5	70–150	< 30
Moderate	1.0–1.5	510	150–200	30–50
Severe	< 1.0	> 10	> 220	> 50

If have associated moderate–severe MR, the peak velocity and transmitral pressure gradients are overestimated so need to calculate valve area. In NSR 60–80 bpm
Adapted from Baumgartner H, et al. J Am Soc Echocardiogr 2009;22:1-23.

What to tell the surgeon:
Pre CPB
- Calcific vs rheumatic valve
- Chordal involvement
- Annulus size (29 ± 4 mm)
- Mitral annular calcification (MAC)
- LA size (severe > 50 mm), LAA thrombus
- RV function, TR severity
Post CPB
- Peak/mean pressure gradients
- Residual MR
- Prosthetic function

Mitral Valve
Mitral Stenosis

Patient with restricted MV leaflet motion from rheumatic MV disease shown during diastole using TEE 3D Zoom from (A) LA side in surgeon's orientation and (B) LV side. (C) 2D TEE ME AV LAX view shows typical hockey stick appearance of AMVL, (D) 2D color Doppler flow acceleration and spectral Doppler high pressure gradient. (E) Reconstructed 3D model shows severe bileaflet restriction and tethering.

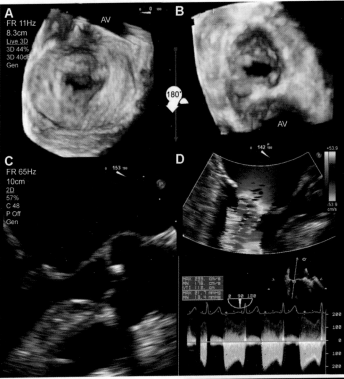

Restricted Mitral Valve

- Thick leaflets, calcium
- No prolapse
- Restricted mobility
- Annular calcium
- Chordal restriction
- Valve replacement

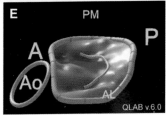

Mitral Valve
Ischemic MR

Ischemic Mitral Regurgitation (MR)
- Common, anterior MI (15%), inferior MI (40%)
- MR severity related to size of wall motion abnormality

Etiologies (based on MV leaflet mobility):
- Normal: annular dilatation ± perforation
- Excessive: prolapse ± flail ± torn chordae ± papillary muscle (PM) rupture
- Restricted: displaced PM ± LV dysfunction

Source: Agricola E, et al. Eur J Echocardiogr 2008;9:207-21.

Pathophysiology Ischemic MR
- Annular dilatation
- ↓ Systolic transmitral pressure
- Apical + posterior displaced PMs
- Altered papillary-annular distance
⇓
Decreased leaflet mobility + malcoaptation
⇓
TEE findings
A. Central MR
B. Dilated LV
C. MV annulus dilated
D. Posterior and apical displaced PM
E. ↓ PM – annular angle
F. Tethering MV leaflet (seagull)

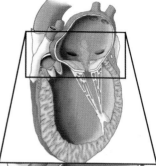

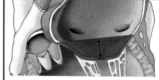

Leaflet tenting is quantified by measuring MV annulus to coaptation point, abnormal if
- Tenting depth (distance) > 0.6 cm
- Tenting area > 1 cm²
- Tenting volume > 2 cm³

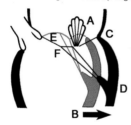

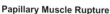

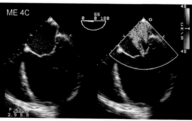

Papillary Muscle Rupture

- 1% of MI, 2–7 days after MI
- Commonly inferior MI, post PM involved
- Partial PM rupture, mobile mass prolapses into LA
- Mitral regurgitation quantification
- ↑ Mortality
- Surgical repair or replacement

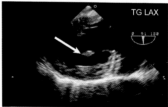

Mitral Valve
Ischemic MR

Patient with restricted MV leaflet motion from ischemic dilated cardiomyopathy shown during systole using RT 3D TEE from the LA side in (A) 3D Live and (B) 3D Zoom. Note the lack of central coaptation (arrows). (C) Compare 2D ME 4C view showing MV leaflet malcoaptation with severe central MR. (D) Reconstructed 3D model shows severe bileaflet restriction, tethering with quantification of tenting volume and height.

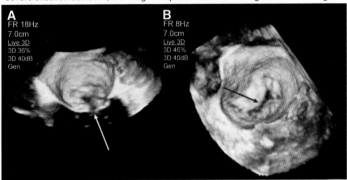

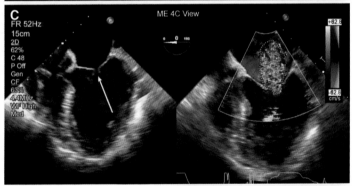

Ischemic Mitral Valve

- Normal leaflet thickness
- Restricted leaflet mobility
- Central leaflet malcoaptation
- Central MR
- Annular dilatation
- Chordal tethering
- Leaflet tenting quantify need for MVR
  - Tenting area > 1 cm^2
  - Tenting volume > 3.9 cm^3

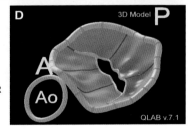

Mitral Valve
MV Repair

MV repair typically involves resection of the abnormal segment, leaflet reconstruction, and insertion of a complete or partial prosthetic ring. This is shown during (A) surgery and (B) systole from the LA side using TEE 3D Zoom. Here the P2 segment is resected and mostly the anterior mitral valve leaflet (AMVL) is seen. Individual sutures can be identified.

3D color Doppler can assess flow through the repaired MV.

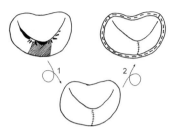

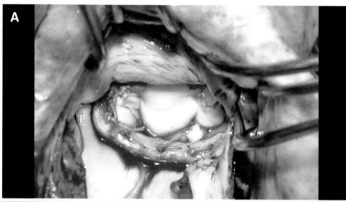

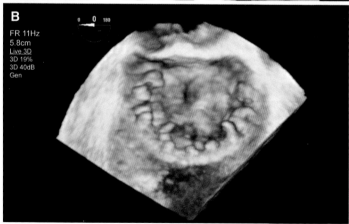

Mitral Valve
Dehisced Mitral Ring

Patient with previous MV repair presents with dehiscence of the partial ring. (A) 2D color compare image shows a gap (arrow) at MV ring with severe MR at the gap and through the valve. (B–D) Series of TEE 3D Zoom images shows the ring from the (B) LA side, (C) LV side with gap from malcoaptation, (D) lateral side is similar to 2D ME AV LAX view and (E) 3D FV color Doppler of MR.

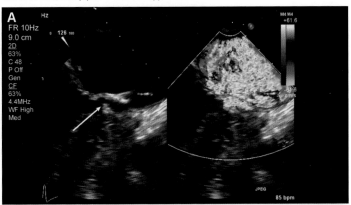

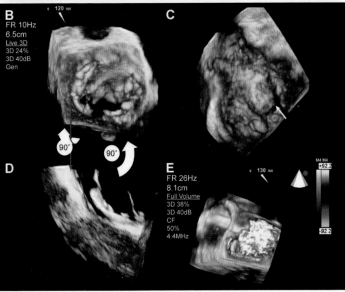

Mitral Valve
MV Quantification

Using a proprietary software package 3D MVQ (QLAB 7.1, Philips Medical Systems) a 3D model of the mitral valve can be constructed as follows:
1. Find and tag the end systolic frame (frame before MV opens).
2. Align MPR and model (place aorta in left side arrow 1D).
   - Blue panel window (1C): red plane through AV, green plane center of MV
   - Green panel window (1A): blue plane through MV annulus
   - Red panel window (1B): blue plane through MV annulus
3. Add reference points on MV annulus (1A for AL + PM, 1B for Ant, Post).
4. Set leaflet nadir (1A or 1B): adjust along minimum line of MV leaflet.
5. Adjust coaptation line (1C) by moving red dots to match ant + post commissures.
6. Move the red diamond to divide the leaflets into three scallops.
7. Position the coaptation point to leaflet coaptation or at the leaflets tips (3).
8. Trace the leaflets (3) while checking the leaflet coaptation on the 3D volume (1C).
9. Find papillary muscle (adjust blue plane), though may not always be possible.

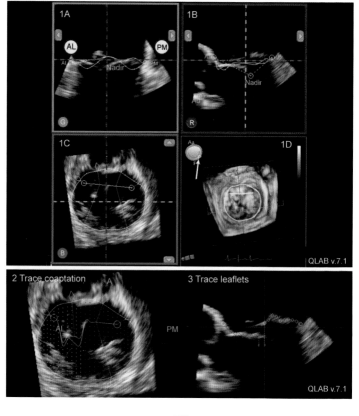

72

Mitral Valve Models

LA Orientation (Fig. A)
1. AL-PM diameter
2. Ant-Post diameter
3. Anterior leaflet length
4. Posterior leaflet length
5. Commissure diameter
6. Annulus perimeter

Anterior Orientation (Figs. B–G)
B. Area posterior leaflet
C. Area anterior leaflet
D. Tenting volume, height
E. Prolapse volume, height
F. Annulus height
G. Aortic-mitral angle

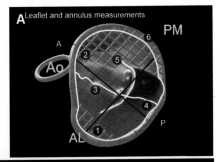

A Leaflet and annulus measurements

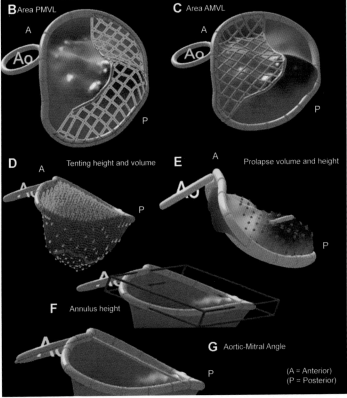

B Area PMVL

C Area AMVL

D Tenting height and volume

E Prolapse volume and height

F Annulus height

G Aortic-Mitral Angle

(A = Anterior)
(P = Posterior)

Mitral Valve
Models

Another proprietary software for MV analysis is 4D-MV Assessment © 2.0 (TomTec Imaging Systems GmbH, Munich, Germany). This is freestanding software that can analyze 3D MV datasets obtained from different vendors. It allows rapid analysis of MV structures, annulus and the leaflet coaptation. It gives a dynamic visualization and quantification of MV morphology and function including (1) prolapse topology, (2) regurgitant orifice, (3) coaptation line and (4) jet origin. This differs from the static model created by 3D MVQ (QLab, Philips Medical System).

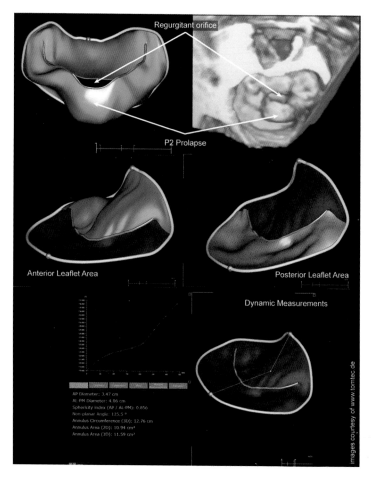

Regurgitant orifice

P2 Prolapse

Anterior Leaflet Area

Posterior Leaflet Area

Dynamic Measurements

AP Diameter: 3.47 cm
AL-PM Diameter: 4.06 cm
Sphericity Index (AP / AL-PM): 0.856
Non-planar Angle: 125.5 °
Annulus Circumference (3D): 12.76 cm
Annulus Area (2D): 10.94 cm²
Annulus Area (3D): 11.59 cm²

images courtesy of www.tomtec.de

Mitral Valve
Models

eSie Valves® (pronounced ez valves) by Siemens is a proprietary software available for MV and AV analysis. It is freestanding software that enables 3D visualization of MV structures, spatial relationships and blood flow. It takes 5–10 min to create a dynamic 3D MV model of a complete heart cycle. (A) There is a streamlined workflow that involves 4 steps: (1) alignment, (2) landmark detection (3) surface detection and (4) summary. The software is semi-automated after the user loads the 3D dataset. The views are automatically extracted, aligned and tracked. The user verifies that the automated landmark with labeling and surface detection is accurate and the modeling is complete. (B) A comprehensive biometric and kinematic measurement suite is available in a numerical, graphical output as well as mapped to the model.

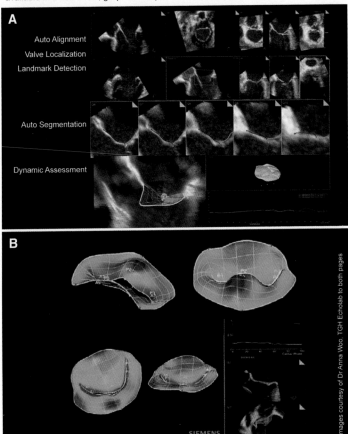

Mitral Valve
Models

A patient with Barlows MV has bileaflet prolapse. (A) This is shown using Siemens MV modeling software in 2D MPR (1) 5C, (2) MV SAX at the annulus level, (3) 2C and (4) parameterized displacement model. (B) The MV model can be superimposed on the 2D image to play dynamically. MV models are also shown as (C) realistic rendering and (D) color coding with solid colors.

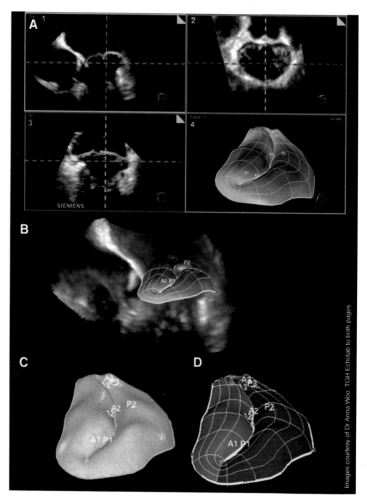

Mitral Valve
Models

A patient with fibroelastic MV disease and a flail P2 segment. (A) This is shown in a 3D 5C view. (B) Using Siemens MV modeling software, a solid color MV model is shown superimposed on the 5C view with prolapse of P2 and plays dynamically. (C) Parameterized displacement and (D) solid color coding MV models are shown from the LA side.

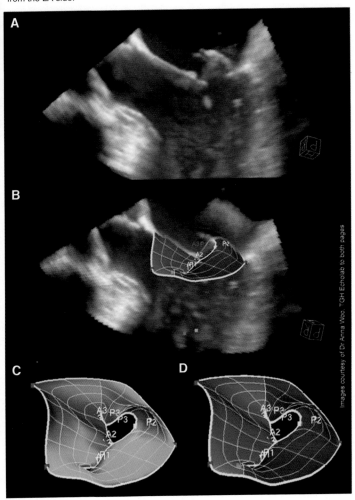

Mitral Valve
3DQ

More accurate assessment of MV leaflet segments can be performed with 2D Multi Planar Reconstruction (MPR) using 3DQ software (Philips Medical Systems) for 3D Zoom and FV MV datasets.

1. (A) Green (ME 5C view) and red (ME MC view) planes are positioned at the center of the MV. Blue plane is aligned parallel to the MV annulus.
2. The blue panel is the MV SAX view and is a reference to display: posterior (PC) and anterior (AC) commissures, left atrial appendage (LAA) and aortic valve (AV).
3. The green plane can be moved posteriorly (B) or anteriorly (C). Different MV segments are displayed in the green panel and are easily identified by looking at the position of the green plane on the blue panel (A). Assessment of individual MV segments for prolapse can be accurately identified.

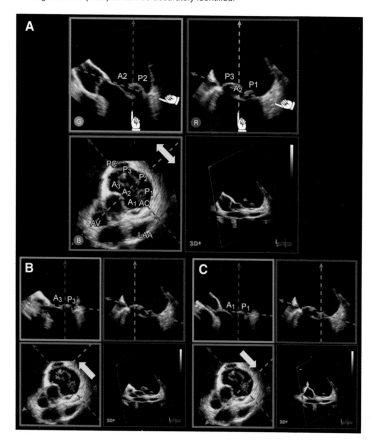

Mitral Valve
Vena Contracta

Vena contracta (VC) size can quantify mitral regurgitant jets in 2D. (A) In 2D TEE the VC width is measured at the narrowest portion of the regurgitant jet immediately distal to the regurgitant orifice. This measurement assumes a round cross section of the regurgitant jet. (B) 3D color Doppler dataset of a MR jet can be exported to 3DQ software (Philips Medical Systems) for measurement of VC area. Shown is a posterior MR jet that hugs the LA wall from the surgeon's orientation.

1. Red and green planes are positioned using the hand cursor parallel to the center of the MR jet (C1 and C2).
2. The blue plane is then moved perpendicular to the green and red planes through the narrowest point of the MR jet just above the regurgitant orifice (C1 and C2).
3. Vena contracta cross section is shown in the blue panel (C3). Vena contracta area (VCA) can be traced and its irregular shape appreciated.

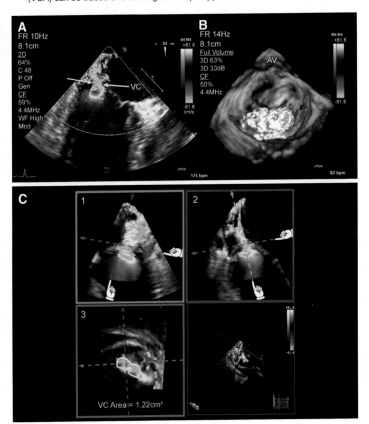

Aortic Valve
Normal Anatomy

Normal Aortic Valve (AV) and Aortic Root Anatomy

The aortic valve is part of the aortic root that includes the aortic annulus, aortic valve cusps, sinuses of Valsalva, sinotubular junction (STJ) and proximal ascending aorta.

There is no true ring-shaped anatomic AV **annulus**; instead it has a crown- shaped base at the aortoventricular junction.

3 valve cusps: Right (most anterior), Non (near IAS), Left (near PA)

Each cusp is comprised of a base, body, and free margin:
- Hinge point is the basal cusp attachment point at the aortoventricular junction.
- Cusp free margin has a central thickened tip and the nodule of Arantius and **lunulae** on either side, which serve as points of cusp coaptation.
- Lambl's excrescences are normal variant degenerative strands on the ventricular side of cusps.

Commissures refer to the area where 2 adjacent cusp margins meet the aorta.

Interleaflet triangles are spaces between the base of the AV cusps that are exposed to ventricular pressures.

Sinuses of Valsalva are 3 ball-shaped outpouches of the aorta that give rise to the coronary ostia (R, L) and are important to AV function.

The upper portions of the sinuses of Valsalva meet the aorta at the nonlinear **sinotubular junction** and forms the superior attachment of the AV cusps.

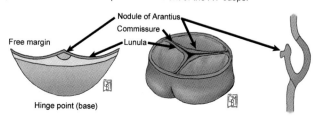

Aortic Root Relationships

Cusps:
Non: AMVL, membranous IVS
Right: membranous IVS, anterior LV
Left: AMVL, anterior LV

Inter-leaflet triangles:
Non/R: RA, RV, TV (septal leaflet)
R/L: potential space aorta and PA
L/non: LA, AMVL

Coronary sinuses of Valsalva:
Non: LA, RA, transverse pericardial
Right: RA, free pericardium
Left: LA, free pericardium

Source: Ho S. Eur J Echocard 2009; 10:i3-10.

Free margin (FM) length = 28–34 mm
Cusp height = 13–16 mm
Cusp base = 42–59 mm (1.5 × FM length)
Cusp area: non > R > L
Hinge point: cusp attach to aorta

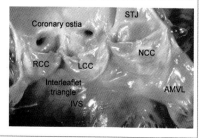

Aortic Valve
2D Assessment

Thin AV cusps make 3D imaging of the AV challenging. Dropout and reverberation artifacts created by heavily calcified or prosthetic valves viewed by 2D imaging will also impede good 3D image quality. However, 3D TEE color Doppler does accurately locate paravalvular leaks for prosthetic valves. Off-line planimetry of the AV, LVOT and vena contracta areas can be performed to grade lesion severity.

xPlane (A) 2D and (B) color Doppler views simultaneously display both ME AV SAX and LAX views in 2 side-by-side panels. Moving the cursor (line) images different cusps in the right display. Shown here are the non (N) and right (R) AV cusps. (B) Despite a low FR (< 10 Hz), xPlane color Doppler is particularly useful when determining the etiology of AI or location of a prosthetic paravalvular leak.

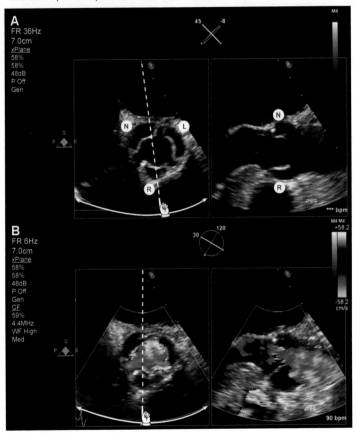

Aortic Valve
3D Assessment

Live 3D obtained from standard 2D views provides real-time information that can help guide percutaneous procedures. To optimize the 3D Live ME (C) SAX or (D) LAX AV views, adjust the gain and use the `lateral steer' function to center the AV. 3D Live ME AV LAX view shows only a portion of the AV even after rotation (arrow). Increasing gain improves cusp definition but obliterates the surrounding structures. 3D TG or deep gastric AV views are rarely used given the poor image definition in comparison to 2D/3D ME and 2D transgastric images.

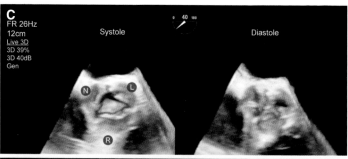

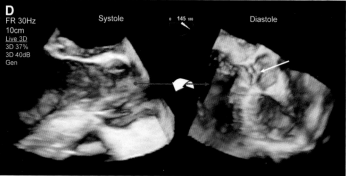

3D Zoom images a greater volume of tissue so it may be more suitable for larger aortic valves and to include part of the aortic root. The frame rate is lower.
1. Begin with either the ME AV SAX or LAX view so the 2D biplane preview shows the entire AV.
2. (E) Position the volume box with adjustment of the x, y, and z axes to enclose the entire AV and aortic root in both SAX and LAX.
3. Initial 3D Zoom acquisition produces an over-gained (brown speckled) uncropped AV SAX (F) or (H) unrotated LAX image.
4. (G, I) Reduce the gain and optimize the image by using the smoothing, brightness, and magnification functions. (G) An initial AV SAX acquisition shows the AV "en face". (I) The LAX acquisition requires rotation to show a tricuspid AV.

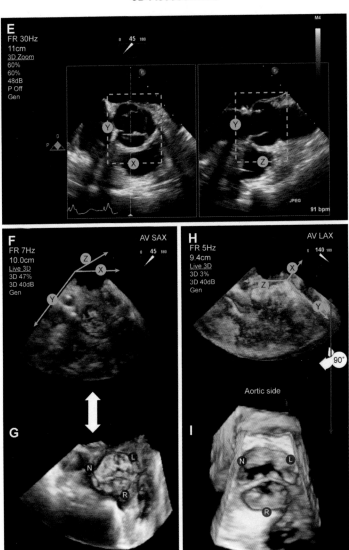

Aortic Valve
3D Assessment

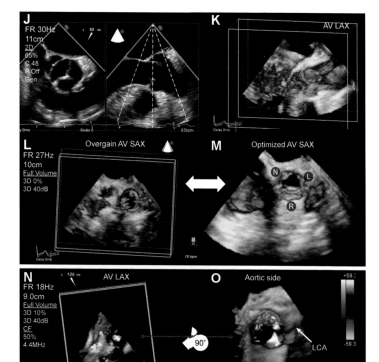

3D Full Volume (FV) has the largest 3D dataset and is useful to image the entire AV, aortic root and LVOT. Compared with 3D Zoom, a higher frame rate improves temporal resolution but the lower spatial resolution provides a less detailed image.
1. 3D FV acquisition begins with optimized 2D ME AV SAX or LAX views.
2. (J) FV acquisition in a 2D preview image is ECG gated (see pg. 12).
3. Initial FV acquisition is displayed (K) with an overlying crop box at 50% cropped AV LAX and (L) over-gained AV SAX views.
4. (M) Adjust gain and optimize the image as described for 3D Zoom AV SAX.
5. The crop box can cut the image in 3 axes using 6 planes or a free plane.

3D FV color Doppler is used in any AV view. (N) Initial FV AV LAX color Doppler gives a 3D image with an overlying crop box. (O) The crop box can be adjusted and the image rotated to view the AV from the aortic side (arrow, left coronary artery).

Aortic Valve
3D Assessment

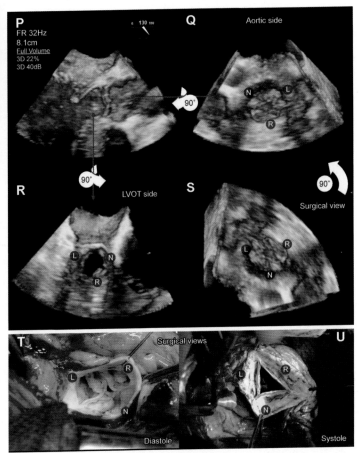

Image Rotation can be performed in any 3D mode using the track ball and Z-rotation function. (P) 3D FV AV LAX is rotated to view the AV from either the (Q) aortic side, (R) LVOT side, or (S) in a surgical orientation. Note the altered position of the AV cusps in the different orientations. (Q) From the aortic orientation, coronary anatomy and aortic root pathology can be identified. (R) From the LVOT orientation the AV is roofed by the AMVL. This view is useful to identify LVOT subvalvular obstruction from septal hypertrophy, membrane, or SAM. (S) Compare the surgical orientation with intraoperative photos (courtesy of Dr C. Feindel) of (T) a normal aortic root in diastole and (U) in systole after resection during an AV sparing root procedure.

Aortic Valve
3D Assessment

eSie Valves® (pronounced ez valves) by Siemens is freestanding software available for MV and AV analysis. It is the only software that constructs patient specific physiologic dynamic 3D AV models. (A) There is a streamlined workflow that involves 4 steps: (1) alignment, (2) landmark detection, (3) surface detection and (4) summary. The software is semi-automated as the views are automatically extracted, aligned and tracked. (B) The user verifies that the automated landmark with labeling and surface detection is accurate and the modeling is complete. (C) The models provide morphological quantification and measurement of dynamic variations. (D) A unique feature is the simultaneous analysis and display of the aortic-mitral complex. (E) Specific measurements include the hinge to ostial distance.

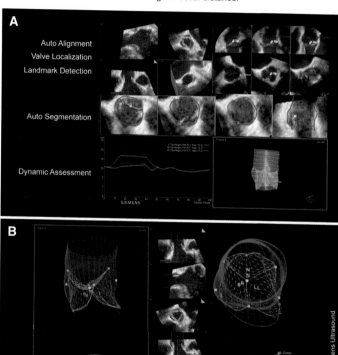

Courtesy of H. Houle, Siemens Ultrasound

Aortic Valve
3D Assessment

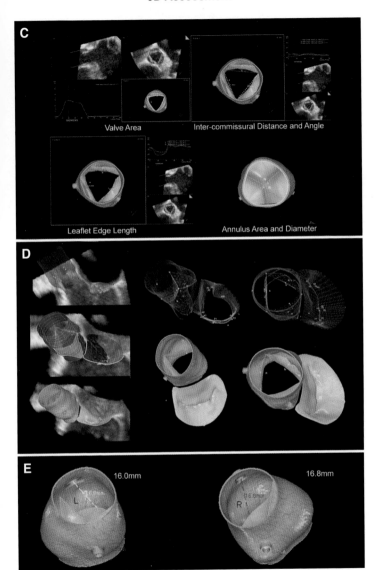

Aortic Valve
Aortic Stenosis

1. Etiology: valvular, subvalvular, supravalvular
   - Valvular: degenerative/calcific, rheumatic, congenital bicuspid
   - Subvalvular: membrane, IHSS, SAM
2. 2D/3D findings:
   - Valvular calcium location, etiology (degenerative vs. rheumatic)
   - Restricted cusp opening
   - SAX: # of cusps (tri vs. bicuspid), planimetry (difficult if calcified)
   - LAX: systolic doming (< 15 mm opening, angle < 90°)
   - Aortic sclerosis: thickened cusps without hemodynamic significance
3. Color Doppler findings:
   - 2D Color: turbulence at level of obstruction
   - 3D Color: limited use
4. 2D spectral Doppler findings:
   - PW: locate level of obstruction
   - CW: peak/mean velocity and pressure gradients varies with flow
     - Underestimate: ↓ LV function, MR, poor Doppler alignment, L→R shunt
     - Overestimate: high CO, AI
     - If LVOT V_{peak} > 1.5 m/s or AV V_{peak} < 3.0 m/s, use modified Bernoulli: peak AS gradient = 4 [(AV velocity peak)^2 – (LVOT velocity peak)^2]
   - CW: continuity equation VTI (LVOT, AV) for AV area
5. Grade stenosis severity (see table below)
6. LVH, small, postero-basal hypokinesis, poor LV underestimates AS
7. Additional features: post-stenotic aortic dilatation, functional MR, MAC

	Valve Area (cm^2)	Indexed Valve Area (cm^2/m^2)	Peak Velocity (m/s)	Pressure Peak (mmHg)	Gradient Mean (mmHg)	
					AHA	ESC
Normal	3.0–4.0		1.4–2.2	8–20		
Mild	> 1.5	> 0.85	2.6–2.9	20–40	< 20	< 30
Mod	1.0–1.5	0.6–0.85	3.0–4.0	40–70	20–40	30–50
Severe	< 1.0	< 0.6	> 4.0	> 70	> 40	> 50

Adapted from Baumgartner H, et al. J Am Soc Echocardiogr 2009;22:1-23.

What to tell the surgeon:
Pre CPB
- Rheumatic, calcific etiology
- Annulus size (for stentless valve: STJ within 10%)
- Calcified AMVL (restricted motion) or aorta (difficult minimal access)
- AV area estimate (prosthetic mismatch), pressure gradients
- Post-stenotic root dilatation, location of coronary ostia
- LVH (concentric), septal hypertrophy (SAM, LVOT diameter)
Post CPB
- Prosthetic valve stability, leaflet mobility
- Paravalvular, valvular leaks
- Peak/mean pressure gradients
- No LVOT obstruction with SAM or VSD (rare)
- Ventricular function (right and left), intra-cavitary gradient (↑ mortality)

Aortic Valve
Aortic Stenosis

Calcific AS gives thickened and immobile cusps as seen in the (A) planimetered 2D ME AV SAX, (B) 3D Live ME AV SAX and (C) 2D ME AV LAX. (C) Turbulence is seen starting at the AV in the 2D AV LAX color compare view. (D) ME AV LAX view, rotation of the FV AV dataset allows it to be viewed from the (E) aortic or (F) LVOT side. (G) Intraoperative photo of calcific aortic stenosis.

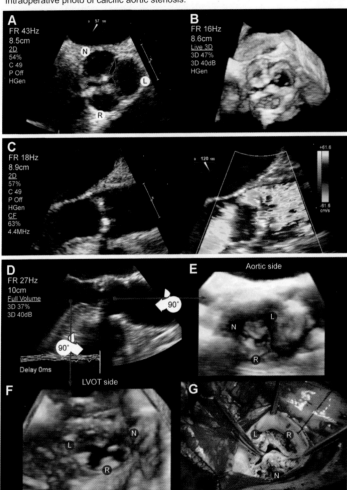

Aortic Valve
Aortic Stenosis Quantification

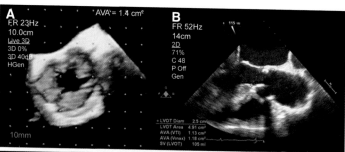

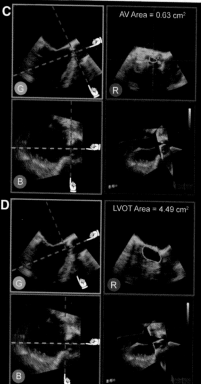

Similar to 2D TEE, accurate on- and off-line AV area planimetry is difficult in calcific AS where the cusp edges are poorly defined and identification of the orifice is difficult.

(A) On-line 3D AV area is crudely estimated by overlying a 10 mm spaced grid.

(B) In 2D TEE the continuity equation estimates a circular LVOT with a similar AV area to planimetry in this example.

(C, D) Off-line planimetry of (C) AV and (D) LVOT areas is performed by importing any 3D dataset into the 3DQ software (Philips Medical System). In this 3D Live AV SAX dataset, the green, blue, and red planes are aligned through the center of the structure and then each area is traced.

This off-line software uses no geometric assumptions. It has provided insight into the non-circular shape of the LVOT. This, in turn, has raised questions over the accuracy of the continuity equation for AV area assessment. A modified form of the continuity equation can be used to calculate AV area where the LV stroke volume is obtained using 3DQA and 2D spectral Doppler is used to obtain the VTI.

Aortic Valve
Rheumatic Aortic Stenosis

Rheumatic valvular disease causes thickening of the cusp edges and commissural fusion. A circular-shaped orifice is seen in the (A) 2D ME AV SAX view and this (B) excised rheumatic AV. The ME AV LAX (C) 2D and (E) rotated 3D FV views show reduced systolic excursion of the thickened cusps. (D) 2D color Doppler shows turbulent flow at the level of the valve.

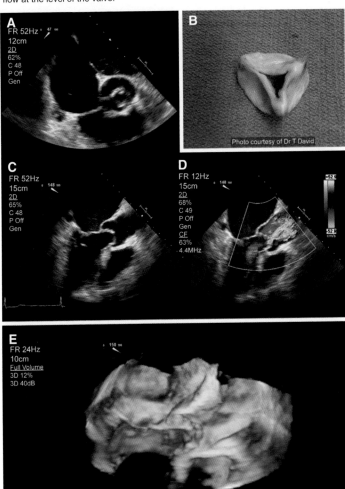

Aortic Valve
Aortic Insufficiency

1. Etiology of insufficiency:
   - Valve: prolapse, calcified, bicuspid, rheumatic, endocarditis
   - Dilated annulus + root: Marfan's, aneurysm, HBP, aortitis
   - Loss of commissural support: trauma, dissection, VSD
2. 2D/3D findings:
   - AV: # cusps, coaptation (SAX, LAX), diastolic fluttering or lack of cusp closure, prolapse, calcified/fused, bicuspid
   - Root dimensions (systole): LVOT, annulus, sinuses, STJ, aorta
3. 2D color Doppler findings (3D color of limited use):
   - Color: diastolic turbulence in LVOT. Jet direction (LAX): central or eccentric. Jet location (SAX): central or commissural
   - Color: measure JH/LVOT (LAX), Jet /LVOT CSA (SAX), vena contracta
4. Spectral Doppler findings:
   - CW: density, diastolic decay measured as PHT or deceleration slope
   - CW: ↑ LVOT velocity > 1.5 m/s
   - PW/CW: diastolic flow reversal in arch/descending/abdominal aorta
   - Calculate ERO area, regurgitant fraction (RF), regurgitant volume (RegV)
5. LV dilated, function variable
6. Associated findings (indirect effect on MV): premature MV closure, reverse doming AMVL, fluttering AMVL, presystolic (diastolic) MR, jet lesion AMVL
7. Severe insufficiency is based on the following findings:
   - Specific: central jet JH/LVOT > 65%, vena contracta > 6 mm
   - Supportive: PHT < 200 ms, abdominal aorta holodiastolic reversal, ↑ LV size
   - Quantitative: RegV > 60 cc, RF > 50%, EROA > 0.3 cm^2

Method	Mild	Moderate	Severe
Jet/LVOT width[a] (%)	< 25	25–64	≥ 65
Jet/LVOT CSA[a] (%)	< 5	5–59	≥ 60
CW density	Faint	Dense	Dense
PHT (ms)	> 500	200–500	< 200
Descending aorta reversal	Early brief	Intermediate	Holodiastolic
Vena contracta[a] (mm)	< 3	3–6	> 6
ERO area (cm^2)	< 0.10	0.1–0.29	≥ 0.30
Regurgitant volume (cc)	< 30	30–59	≥ 60
Regurgitant fraction (%)	20–30	30–49	≥ 50

[a]Nyquist limit 50–60 cm/s
Adapted from Zoghbi W et al. J Am Soc Echocardiogr 2003;16:777-802

What to tell the surgeon:
Pre CPB
- Root vs. valve pathology, dimensions of aortic root
- Number, morphology, and coaptation of cusps (prolapse), calcified cusps
- Location + direction AI (central, eccentric commissural), AI severity
- Pulmonary valve annulus size (within 10–15% of aortic annulus for Ross)
- ±PI, R/O fenestrations (for Ross procedure)
Post CPB
- Cusp coaptation above the annular plane (LAX)
- Location and severity of AI

Aortic Valve
Aortic Insufficiency

Color Doppler
Assesses jet direction and AI severity by measuring jet area or height. Jet distance into the LV relies on hemodynamics and ultrasound machine settings; thus it is a poor measure of AI severity. Nyquist limit is 50–60 cm/s.
(A) Jet height (JH) to LVOT height is measured in ME AV LAX view.
(B) Jet area to LVOT area is measured below the AV cusps in the ME AV SAX view.

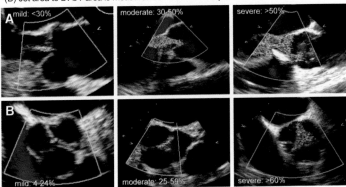

Spectral Doppler Tracings
(A) CW Trace: TG LAX or deep TG, assess density (compare with inflow), steepness, slope. Best alignment occurs if peak initial gradient is > 40 mmHg (V > 300 cm/s).
(B) PW Trace: holodiastolic flow in the proximal arch (see below) and descending aorta is specific but not sensitive for severe AI. The more distal within the descending aorta, the greater the AI severity.

CW weak density	CW moderate density	CW dense density
Mild - "flat top"	Moderate - ↑ angle	Severe - steep slope
Decay slope < 2 m/s	Decay slope 2–3.5 m/s	Decay slope > 3 m/s
PHT > 500 ms	PHT 200–500 ms	PHT < 200 ms

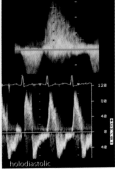

93

Aortic Valve
Aortic Insufficiency

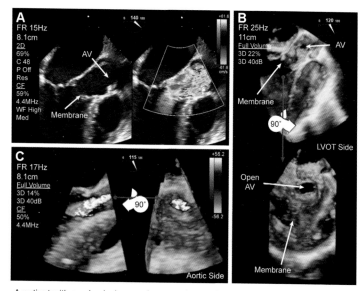

A patient with a subvalvular membrane and central AI from cusp malcoaptation. The subvalvular shelf is seen in ME AV LAX (A) 2D color compare, (B) 3D FV and rotated to the LVOT side. (C) 3D color Doppler ME AV LAX and rotated to the aortic side demonstrates central AI.

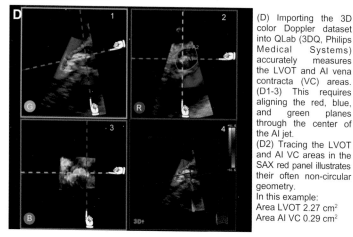

(D) Importing the 3D color Doppler dataset into QLab (3DQ, Philips Medical Systems) accurately measures the LVOT and AI vena contracta (VC) areas. (D1-3) This requires aligning the red, blue, and green planes through the center of the AI jet.
(D2) Tracing the LVOT and AI VC areas in the SAX red panel illustrates their often non-circular geometry.
In this example:
Area LVOT 2.27 cm^2
Area AI VC 0.29 cm^2

Aortic Valve
Unicuspid

Estimated unicuspid AV incidence is 0.02%. Results from failure of 2 commissures to develop during valvulogenesis creating a central or eccentrically placed orifice.

2 types - Unicommissural > acommisssural depending on whether there is lateral attachment to the aorta at the valve orifice level.

(A) Unicommissural Single cusp attaches laterally to aorta and wraps around to create the valve orifice.
(B) Acommissural Centrally placed orifice with 3 surrounding raphe ridges.

There is maldevelopment of all 3 cusps with no commissures or lateral aortic wall attachment. During diastole, the raphe may form the 'Mercedes Benz' sign and thus the valve may be mistaken for tricuspid. However, during systole, the valve orifice is 'tear drop' shaped instead of the normal triangle.

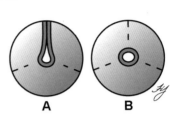

A   **B**

Unicuspid valves are often heavily calcified with AS being more common than mixed AV disease. Associated aortic dilatation has been reported although at lower frequency than for bicuspid disease.

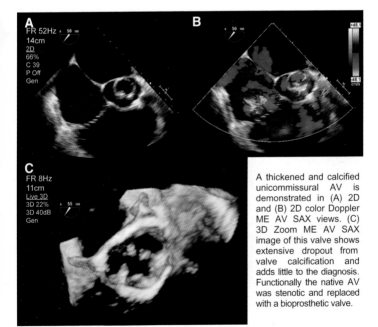

A thickened and calcified unicommissural AV is demonstrated in (A) 2D and (B) 2D color Doppler ME AV SAX views. (C) 3D Zoom ME AV SAX image of this valve shows extensive dropout from valve calcification and adds little to the diagnosis. Functionally the native AV was stenotic and replaced with a bioprosthetic valve.

Aortic Valve
Bicuspid

Bicuspid Aortic Valve (BAV)
2 cusps:
    Congenital: equal or unequal (usually anterior > posterior) cusp size
    Acquired: unequal cusp size from fused commissure
    Describe commissure location (i.e. 4 + 10 o'clock), anterior/posterior, right/left
    Raphe present at 90° to commissural opening
Thickened aortic cusps (may be mild)
Systolic elliptical orifice opening (SAX view)
Systolic cusp doming (LAX view)
Eccentric diastolic closure line (LAX)
Diastolic doming from cusp prolapse (LAX)
Usually have 3 sinuses of Valsalva
Left ventricular hypertrophy (LVH)
Location of coronary ostia (usually 180° apart)
    Type 1: 2 coronary arteries anterior to valve orifice
    Type 2: valve orifice separates the coronaries
Associated pathology: AI, PDA, VSD
    Aortopathy: dilatation, aneurysm, dissection
    Coarctation of aorta in 15–20% BAV; 80–85% of coarcts have BAV

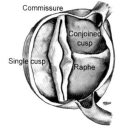

Bicuspid Aortic Valve LAX
Normal AV cusps open and close in the center of the sinuses of Valsalva. Bicuspid AV cusp opening is frequently eccentric and the cusps appear domed during systole (arrow) from incomplete opening, ME AV LAX (A) 3D Live and (B) 2D views. The diastolic coaptation line may appear eccentric with prolapse of the cusp body (diastolic doming), ME AV LAX (C) 3D Live and (D) 2D.

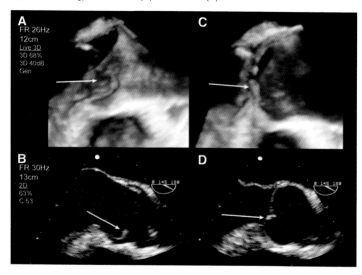

Aortic Valve
Bicuspid

Bicuspid Aortic Valve SAX

It is best to determine the number of AV cusps during systole in the ME AV SAX view. (A) In a normal AV with 3 cusps, the opened orifice is triangular. (B) The orifice is oval or "fish mouthed" in appearance with a bicuspid valve. During diastole a bicuspid valve raphe (D) may form the "Mercedes Benz" sign similar to a normal AV (C).

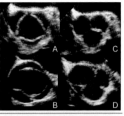

TEE ME AV SAX views show a bicuspid valve using (A) 2D color compare and (B) 3D Zoom. Note the commissures at 1 and 7 o'clock, thickened cusps, restricted opening, and turbulent flow associated with aortic stenosis. There is corresponding dropout from shadowing that occurs in both 2D and 3D. (C) This patient also had a dilated aortic root and ascending aorta aneurysm in 3D Live ME AV LAX view.

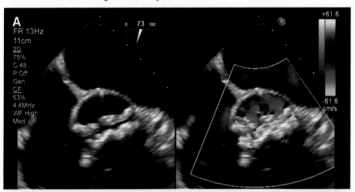

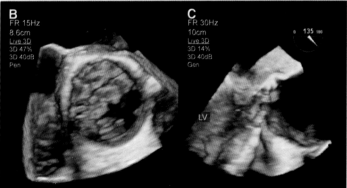

Aortic Valve
Sinus of Valsalva Aneurysm

(A) Non-coronary sinus of Valsalva aneurysm with color flow is demonstrated in the 2D ME AV SAX color compare view. The characteristic windsock deformity expands in systole. (B) 3D FV ME view images the windsock from the surgeon's orientation as shown in (C). (D) The orifice of the windsock (arrow) is shown in this rotated FV ME view. (E) 3D color Doppler demonstrates flow into the windsock and RA (arrow).

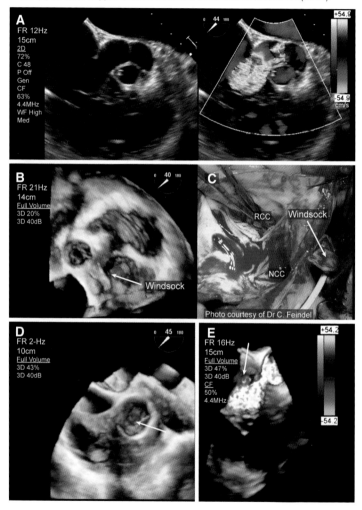

Aortic Valve
Sinus of Valsalva Aneurysm

Right sinus of Valsalva aneurysm with windsock deformity seen in (A) 2D xPlane ME AV LAX and SAX views. (B) 3D FV ME AV LAX and rotated to the aortic side better shows the entire windsock orifice (arrows). The orifice is also demonstrated in the rotated 3D FV (C) ME RVOT view and (D) base of the heart view. (E) Rupture of the windsock into the RV is shown by 2D color Doppler xPlane ME AV LAX and SAX.

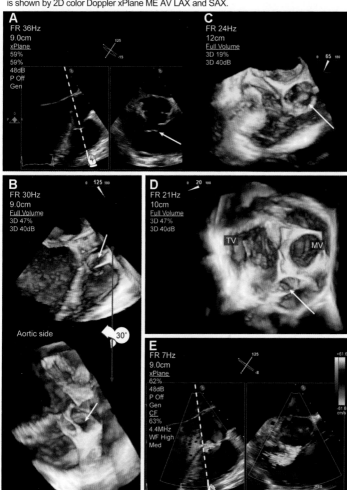

Tricuspid Valve
Normal

Tricuspid Valve Anatomy
- Annulus: fibrous ring
  Leaflets attach at hinge point
  Apically displaced below MV annulus (4C view)
  Distensible size
  - Diameter end-systole 28 mm ± 5
  - TV area 7–9 cm^2
- 3 Valve leaflets: (size varies)
  Septal (S) > anterior (A) > posterior (P)
- 3 Commissures:
  - Anteroseptal, anteroposterior, posteroseptal
- Chordae: support leaflets during systole,
  attach to papillary muscles and directly to septal
  wall (unlike MV)
- 3 Papillary muscles:
  - Anterior, posterior, ± septal

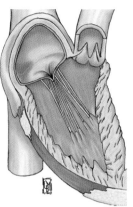

2D TEE Tricuspid Valve Views

Coronary Sinus (CS) view (0°)
(posterior/left, septal/right)
Advance probe from ME 4C view to GE
junction, see TV and inflow from CS

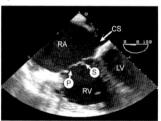

Modified Bicaval view (110–140°)
(posterior/left, anterior/right)
Increase angle from 90° bicaval view,
TV centered, good Doppler alignment

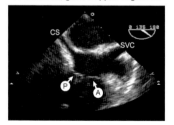

ME 4C view (0°)
(anterior or posterior/left, septal/right)
Annulus dimensions (ES 28 ± 5 mm)
TR direction + trace extent into RA

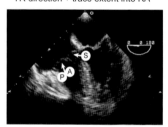

ME RV Inflow-Outflow view (60–75°)
(posterior/left, anterior or septal/right)
TR jet is often seen and better aligned
to spectral Doppler

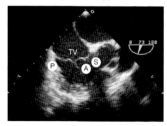

Tricuspid Valve
Normal

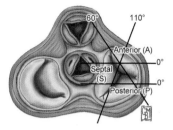

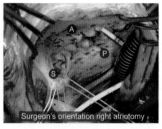

3D TEE imaging of the TV is difficult due to its anterior location and thin leaflets. This results in echo dropout of normal TV leaflets. 2D or 3D transthoracic echocardiography is better able to view anterior cardiac structures. Off-line planimetry using 3D datasets can be performed to quantify TV area.

xPlane (A) Color Doppler ME RVOT and (B) 2D TG views simultaneously display 2 TV views in side-by-side panels. Positioning of the cursor line allows rotation around the entire TV from the ME and TG views with accurate identification of each leaflet.

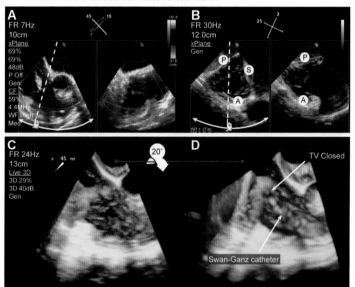

Live 3D from standard 2D views provides real-time information. The normal TV is difficult to image due to its thin leaflets and distance from the probe. (C) To optimize the 3D Live ME RVOT view of the TV, increase gain and use the 'lateral steer' function to center the valve. (D) More of the TV is displayed by tilting the image downward.

Tricuspid Valve
3D Assessment

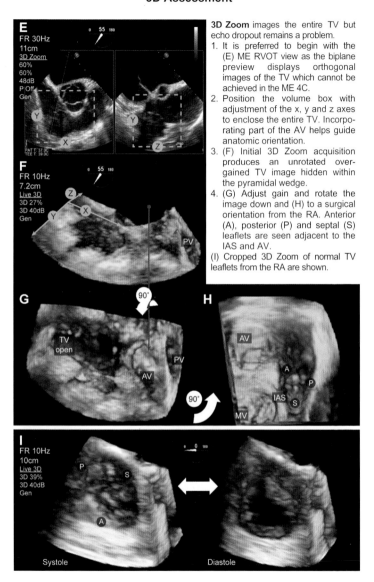

3D Zoom images the entire TV but echo dropout remains a problem.

1. It is preferred to begin with the (E) ME RVOT view as the biplane preview displays orthogonal images of the TV which cannot be achieved in the ME 4C.
2. Position the volume box with adjustment of the x, y and z axes to enclose the entire TV. Incorporating part of the AV helps guide anatomic orientation.
3. (F) Initial 3D Zoom acquisition produces an unrotated over-gained TV image hidden within the pyramidal wedge.
4. (G) Adjust gain and rotate the image down and (H) to a surgical orientation from the RA. Anterior (A), posterior (P) and septal (S) leaflets are seen adjacent to the IAS and AV.

(I) Cropped 3D Zoom of normal TV leaflets from the RA are shown.

Tricuspid Valve
3D Assessment

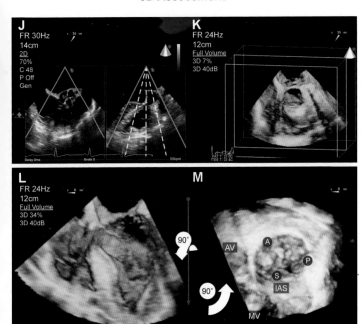

3D Full Volume (FV) results in a larger pyramidal wedge which incorporates more of the surrounding valvular and ventricular structures. The higher frame rate improves temporal resolution. Spatial resolution of the TV is more detailed compared to the other 3D modes.

1. 3D FV acquisition begins with optimized 2D ME 4C or RVOT views.
2. (J) FV acquisition in a preview image is ECG gated over consecutive heartbeats. Shown is ECG (4 beats) FV acquisition from the RVOT view.
3. (K) Initial FV acquisition gives an over-gained (brown speckled) image displayed at 50% cropped with an overlying crop box.
4. Reduce gain and optimize the image by using the smoothing, magnification and brightness functions.
5. The crop box can cut the image in any of the 3 axes using 6 planes of the cropping box or a free plane.

Image Rotation can be performed in any 3D mode using the track ball and Z rotation function. (L) FV ME 4C is cropped and the image is adjusted to show a more detailed TV. (M) Z-Rotation (90°) of the 3D dataset to the surgeon's orientation through a right atriotomy positions the MV at the bottom of the display with the aortic valve (AV) at 9 o'clock. Compare TV leaflets with the surgical view on pg. 101 and to the unrotated 3D Zoom (H and I, pg. 102) image.

Tricuspid Valve
Tricuspid Regurgitation

1. Etiology of regurgitation:
   - Physiological TR > 90% of patients
   - Annulus: dilated, high PAP (MS, MR, Eisenmenger's, cor pulmonale)
   - Valvular: prolapse, rheumatic, carcinoid, myxomatous, endocarditis
     – Carcinoid: thickened, shortened immobile leaflets
     – Rheumatic: TR is more common than TS
   - Ebstein's anomaly: TV leaflets (septal) apically displaced
   - Catheter, pacer
2. 2D/3D findings:
   - Leaflets: thickened, calcified, prolapse, malcoaptation, flail
   - Annulus: dilated > 34 mm end-systole (normal < 28 mm)
3. 2D Doppler findings (3D color of limited use):
   - Color: turbulent (mosaic) retrograde flow, jet direction is usually toward IAS
     laminar (red) retrograde flow if severe RV failure
   - Color: area, vena contracta (proximal jet width), PISA radius
   - CW: systolic flow toward transducer, peak velocity unrelated to TR severity
   - PW: hepatic vein flow systolic reversal is 80% sensitive
   - PW: TV inflow ↑ E wave velocity > 1 m/s
4. Associated findings:
   - RA, RV dilated
   - Paradoxical IVS motion (volume overload), IAS bulges to left "D" shape
   - Dilated IVC (> 2 cm) and hepatic vein (> 1 cm)
5. Regurgitation severity:
   - Color map area for central jet, not valid with eccentric jets
   - Hepatic vein systolic flow reversal, may be absent in chronic TR if RA dilated
   - IVC > 2 cm, no respiratory variation, normal IVC if acute TR
   - CW density and contour: dense triangular with early peaking is severe

Tricuspid Regurgitation Severity

	Mild	Moderate	Severe
RV/RA/IVC size	Normal	Normal or dilated	Dilated
Jet area (cm^2)[a,c]	< 5	5–10	> 10
VC width (cm)[a]	Not defined	Not defined, but < 0.7	> 0.7
PISA (cm)[b]	≤ 0.5	0.6–0.9	> 0.9
CW jet density	Soft, parabolic	Dense, variable shape	Dense, triangular
Hepatic vein flow	S dominance	S blunting	S reversal

Nyquist limit: [a](50–60 cm/s), [b](28 cm/s); [c]not valid with eccentric jets; S = systolic
Adapted from Zoghbi W et al. J Am Soc Echocardiogr 2003;16:777-802.

What to tell the surgeon:
- Leaflet morphology: myxomatous, prolapse, endocarditis
- Annulus size in systole (28 ± 5 mm)
- TR jets number and direction, severity (color map area/ RA area)
Post CPB
- Annulus size
- TR severity
- TV inflow (? stenosis)

104

Tricuspid Valve
TV Perforation and Prolapse

(A) 2D ME 4C color Doppler image displays an echogenic structure traversing the TV associated with severe TR directed toward the IAS. (B)   Intraoperatively, a previously inserted pacemaker wire (arrow) was found to have perforated the anterior TV leaflet causing the TR. (C) Rotating down a 3D Live ME 4C demonstrates the wire (arrow) piercing the anterior leaflet.

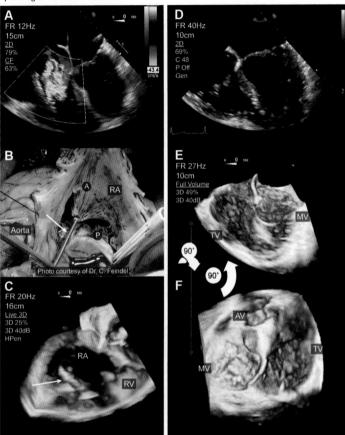

(D–F) This patient with severe TR and MR from multi-segment prolapse underwent a MV replacement and TV repair. (D) 2D ME 4C view demonstrates the thickened and shaggy appearance of the TV and MV. These features are greatly enhanced in 3D FV ME 4C views (E) cropped unrotated and (F) rotated down with z-rotation to show the base of the heart with the AV at the top of the display.

Tricuspid Valve
Tricuspid Stenosis

1. Etiology of stenosis:
   - Valvular: rheumatic (+mitral), carcinoid (+pulmonic)
   - Obstruction: tumor, vegetation, thrombus, extra-cardiac compression
2. 2D/3D findings:
   - Leaflets: thickened
   - Decreased leaflet mobility, tethered leaflet tips (diastolic doming)
3. 2D color Doppler findings (3D color Doppler is of limited use):
   - 2D color: turbulent diastolic flow, also TR (systolic flow)
   - CW: HR between 70–80, TV inflow peak E velocity > 1.0 m/s
     − Mean pressure gradient: mild < 2 mmHg, moderate 2–5 mmHg, > 5 mmHg
   - CW for PHT of TV area (TVA)
4. Associated findings: RA enlarged, IVC dilated (> 2.3 cm)
5. Stenosis severity (severe), ASE guidelines*
   - TV area < 1.0 cm^2
   - Peak velocity > 1.5 m/s, mean pressure > 5 mmHg, VTI > 60 cm
   - PHT valve area is not validated (use TVA = 190/PHT), continuity, PISA

*Source: Baumgartner H, et al. J Am Soc Echocardiogr 2009;22:1-23.

An abnormally thickened and non-calcified TV with greater echogenicity is displayed during systole in (A) 2D ME RVOT view and (B) 3D Zoom in the surgeon's orientation. (C) Surgical photo of a TV repair with a ring. (D) Previous TV repair shows turbulent antegrade diastolic flow with PISA formation in a ME 4C view.

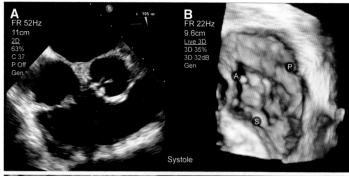

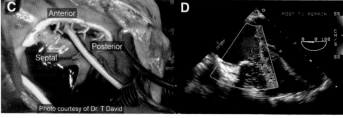

Tricuspid Valve
Rheumatic

Rheumatic valve disease causes leaflet thickening and fusion of the leaflet tips. This patient presented with rheumatic TV, MV and AV disease. (A, B) 2D ME 4C views zoomed on the TV demonstrates the typical appearance of (A) diastolic doming and (B) reverse systolic doming. (C) RA dilatation with chamber smoke is viewed in 2D zoom preview ME views at 45° and 135°. (D) 2D ME 4C color Doppler shows flow turbulence through the stenotic TV and MV. (E) An excised TV leaflet is shown. (F) Rotated 3D FV ME 4C gives an atrial view of the smooth thickened bright TV and MV with reduced diastolic orifices. (G) Mechanical MV and bioprosthetic TV replacements are seen open during diastole from the atria in the rotated 3D FV ME 4C view.

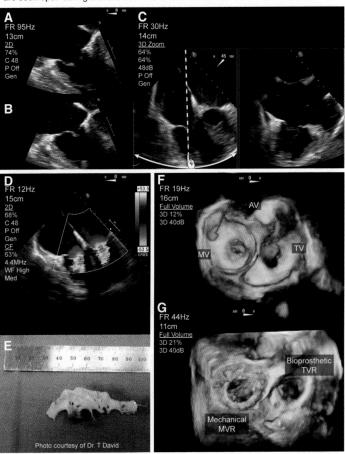

Pulmonic Valve
Normal Anatomy

Pulmonic Valve Anatomy
- Anterior cardiac structure
- Difficult to image with TEE
- Valve: 3 semi-lunar cusps:
  right (R), left (L), anterior (A)
- PA: slightly dilated forming sinus
- AV and PV normally lie at 90° planes
  to each other. ME RVOT view images
  AV SAX with PV in LAX. In the ME AV
  LAX view, the PV is in SAX although it
  is difficult to see as it is anterior.

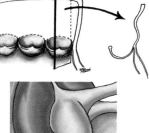

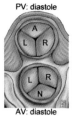
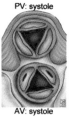

Pulmonic Valve TEE Views

ME RV Inflow-Outflow view (45–60°)
Difficult to see cusps, try zoomed view
Measure PV annulus: 21 ± 3 mm

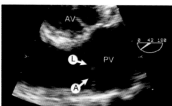

ME Ascending Aortic SAX view (0°)
Useful for Doppler alignment of PA flow
Diameter main PA: 20 ± 5 mm

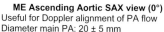
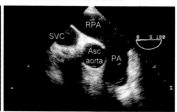

UE Aortic Arch SAX view (60–90°)
Cusp morphology, measure annulus
Doppler alignment for PV or PA flow

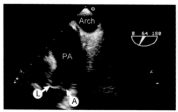

TG RV modified view (30–60°)
Useful Doppler alignment
Normal PV peak velocity 0.5–1.0 m/s

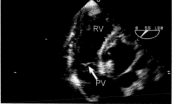

108

Pulmonic Valve
2D and 3D Assessment

3D TEE imaging of the PV is notoriously difficult due to its thin cusp structure and located furthest from the ultrasound beam. Proximity of the PV to the chest facilitates better visualization by transthoracic or epicardial imaging.

xPlane positioning of the line cursor in 2D and color Doppler images allow rotation around the PV and main pulmonary artery (MPA) which are displayed in 2 side-by-side panels. xPlane UE aortic arch (A) 2D with (B) color Doppler shows trace PI. ME ascending aorta (C) 2D with (D) color Doppler views are shown.

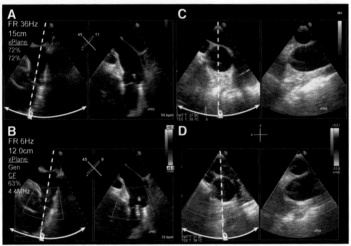

Live 3D can be performed from any standard view and provides real–time information. To optimize the 3D Live ME (E) RVOT and (F) ascending aorta SAX views, adjust the gain and center the PV by using the `lateral steer' function. The PV is incompletely imaged using 3D Live.

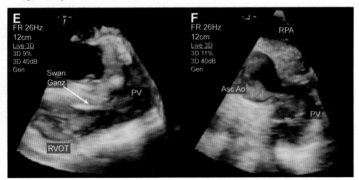

Pulmonic Valve
3D Assessment

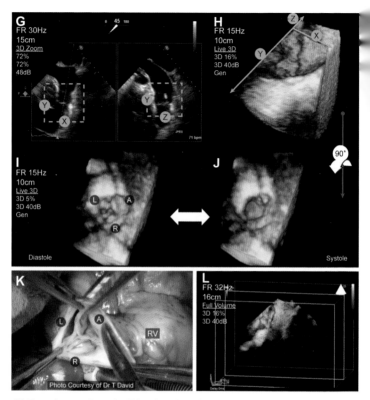

3D Zoom images the entire PV and portions of the RVOT and PA.
1. Begin in the UE arch SAX view which brings the PV closest to the probe.
2. (G) Place a volume box and adjust the x, y, and z axes to enclose the entire PV.
3. (H) Initial zoom acquisition is an unrotated over-gained PV image from the side.
4. (I, J) Rotate the image to view the PV from above in the MPA in the surgeon's orientation (K). Reduce gain and optimize the image using the smoothing, brightness and magnification functions.

3D Full Volume (FV) despite the largest 3D dataset, spatial resolution is not improved and details of the normal PV are difficult to see.
1. 3D FV acquisition begins with optimized 2D UE Arch SAX or ME RVOT views.
2. FV acquisition in a preview image is ECG gated.
3. (L) Initial FV acquisition is an over-gained (brown speckled) image displayed with an overlying crop box and at 50% cropped.
4. Reduce gain and optimize the image as described above. The crop box can cut the image in any of the 3 axes using 6 planes or a free plane.

Pulmonic Valve
Insufficiency and Stenosis

Pulmonic Insufficiency (PI)
1. Etiology of insufficiency:
   - Physiologic PI in 80% patients
   - Valvular: myxomatous, congenital, Marfan's, endocarditis, prosthetic
   - Dilated PA, RVOT, ↑ PA pressures
   - Carcinoid

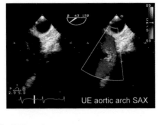

UE aortic arch SAX

2. 2D/3D findings:
   - Difficult to see cusps well as PV is an anterior structure
   - PV annulus or PA dilated
3. 2D Doppler findings (3D color Doppler is of limited use):
   - Color: blue or turbulent diastolic flow in RVOT, may be brief duration
   - PW/CW: diastolic flow away from baseline, density, and deceleration slope
   - PW PV flow: ↑ peak systolic velocity, compare with systemic (AV) flow
4. Associated findings: RV dilated, posterior displacement of LV septum
5. Severity of PI is difficult to quantify
   - Mild PI is normal, Swan-Ganz only causes mild PI
   - Color/spectral Doppler holo-diastolic flow reversal in main PA

Source: Zoghbi W et al. J Am Soc Echocardiogr 2003;16:777-802.

Pulmonic Stenosis (PS)
1. Etiology of stenosis:
   - Normal pulmonic valve area 2 cm^2/m^2
   - Valvular: rheumatic, carcinoid, prosthetic
   - Congenital
   - Infundibular (RV hypertrophy)

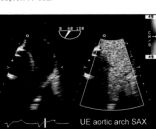

UE aortic arch SAX

2. 2D/3D findings:
   - Valve: thickened, calcified, immobile, systolic doming
   - RVOT narrowed in infundibular PS
   - RVH > 5 mm thick (pressure over-load), RV dilated
   - Post-stenotic PA dilatation (> 20 mm)
3. 2D Doppler findings (3D color Doppler of limited use):
   - Color: turbulent systolic flow at level of obstruction, also may have PI
   - PW to locate level of obstruction (valvular, subvalvular)
   - CW velocity and peak pressure gradients (overestimate if PI),
     - Mild: < 3 m/s, < 36 mmHg
     - Moderate: 3–4 m/s, 36–64 mmHg
     - Severe: > 4 m/s, > 64 mmHg
   - PASP does not equal RVSP in the presence of PS
     - PASP = RVSP (from TR + RAP) - PV pressure gradient
4. Stenosis severity (severe PS by ASE guidelines*)
   - Peak velocity > 4 m/s
   - Peak gradient > 64 mmHg
   - Continuity equation for valve area (< 0.5 cm^2)

Source: Baumgartner H, et al. J Am Soc Echocardiogr 2009;22:1-23.

4

Cardiac Prosthetic Valves

A. Vegas et al., *Real-Time Three-Dimensional Transesophageal* 113
Echocardiography, DOI 10.1007/978-1-4614-0665-5_4,
© Springer Science+Business Media, LLC 2012

Prosthetic Valves
Overview

Types of Prosthetic Valves

Tissue (Bioprosthetic)	**Mechanical**
Stented porcine: Hancock, CE, Mosaic	Caged Ball: Starr-Edwards
Stented bovine: Ionescu-Shiley, CE	Tilting disc: Bjork-Shiley, Medtronic-Hall
Stentless porcine: SPV, Freestyle	Bileaflet: St. Jude, CarboMedics
Homograft: aortic, mitral	Valved conduit: St. Jude, Medtronic-Hall

Normal Prosthetic Valve Findings

Aortic homograft	Antegrade flow similar to native valve
	Thickened aortic annulus/root, no acoustic shadow
	None to trivial valve regurgitation
Tissue valve	Antegrade flow similar to native valve
	3 struts, acoustic shadow
	Mild valvular regurgitation
Caged ball	Antegrade flow through valve periphery
	To avoid cage acoustic shadowing image in LAX
	None to trivial valve regurgitation around "ball"
Tilting disc	Antegrade flow through 2 orifices (major and minor)
	Single disc, acoustic shadowing
	2 to 3 regurgitant washing jets: large central + smaller peripheral
Bileaflet	Antegrade flow through 3 orifices
	Bileaflet motion, acoustic shadowing
	3 regurgitant washing jets: 1 central and 2 peripheral

Prosthetic Valve Pressure Gradients (PG)

Type	Mitral			Aortic[a]		
	Vmax (m/s)	Pmax (mmHg)	Pmean (mmHg)	Vmax (m/s)	Pmax (mmHg)	Pmean (mmHg)
Starr-Edwards	1.9 ± 4	14 ± 5	5 ± 2	3.2 ± 6	38 ± 11	23 ± 88
St. Jude[a]	1.6 ± .3	10 ± 3	4 ± 1	2.4 ± .3	25 ± 5	12 ± 6
Bjork-Shiley	1.6 ± .3	10 ± 2	3 ± 2	2.5 ± 6	23 ± 8	14 ± 5
CE	1.8 ± 2	12 ± 3	6 ± 2	2.5 ± .5	23 ± 8	14 ± 5
Hancock	1.5 ± 3	9 ± 3	4 ± 2	2.4 ± .4	23 ± 7	11 ± 2
Stentless	None	None	None	2.2	19	3 ± 1

- [a]PG varies with valve size (aortic position): 19 mm (20 mmHg), 23 mm (12 mmHg)
- Pressure recovery overestimates St. Jude AVR gradient
- Valve sizes describe the outer valve diameter, not the internal orifice diameter
- Prosthesis patient mismatch: normal prosthesis function with high transvalvular gradient, common in aortic position

What to tell the surgeon post CPB:
- Valve well seated
- Leaflets mobile (2D and color Doppler)
- Valvular functional leaks (washing jets, physiologic)
- Paravalvular leaks (color Doppler)
- Peak and mean valve pressure gradients
- Effective orifice area (aortic valve)
- Obstruction LVOT (MV strut), SAM of AMVL (if AV prosthesis too small)

Prosthetic Valves
Overview

Mechanical Valves		
Valve Type	**Flow Through Valve**	**Echocardiographic Findings**
Starr-Edwards (discontinued 2007) 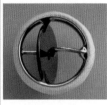 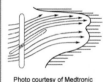 Photo courtesy of Edwards Lifesciences Irvine, California		**Ball Cage** • Ball larger than orifice • Turbulent antegrade flow through valve periphery • High profile • Small orifice, high Pressure • ↑ Thromboembolism risk • Trivial valve regurgitation • No washing jets
Medtronic-Hall (below), Bjork-Shiley (discontinued) 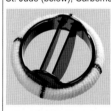 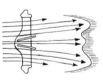 Photo courtesy of Medtronic		**Tilting Disc** • Single disc + eccentric strut/hinge • Opening angle 60–70° • Backpressure on larger disc portion closes disc • 2 antegrade flow orifices across valve (major, minor) • 3 washing jets; large central jet + smaller jets around occluding disc and sewing ring
St. Jude (below), Carbomedics 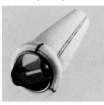 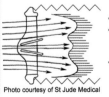 Photo courtesy of St Jude Medical		**Bileaflet** • 2 symmetrical leaflets + 2 hinges, low profile • Bileaflet pivot motion, opens to 80° • Antegrade flow via 3 orifices • Lowest pressure • 3 regurgitant washing jets; 1 central + 2 peripheral • Most regurgitant fraction (10%)
St. Jude (below), Medtronic-Hall Photo courtesy of St Jude Medical		**Valved Conduit** • Typically mechanical valve attached to Dacron conduit • Sewn in as single unit • Cannot have paravalvular leak, as all leaks would appear outside the heart • Washing jets depend on valve type

Prosthetic Valve
Mechanical Prosthesis

(A) Mechanical bileaflet prosthetic valve is comprised of 2 symmetrical leaflets suspended on 2 hinges that allow pivot motion. (B) Pressure opens the leaflets to 80° with antegrade flow through 3 orifices and backpressure closes the leaflets. Shown in the mitral position using TEE in (C) 2D and (D) 3D Live. (E) Washing (regurgitant) jets at the 4 hinge points prevent blood stasis shown using 3D color Doppler. This type of prosthetic valve is typically inserted in the anti-anatomical (perpendicular to native MV commissures) to facilitate opening and minimize submitral chordal entrapment. Patient with MVR St. Jude shown using 3D Zoom during (F) diastole and (G) systole from the LA in the surgeon's orientation.

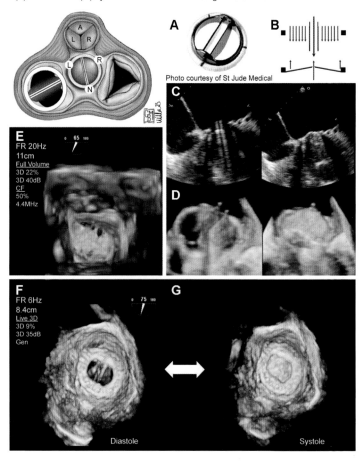

Photo courtesy of St Jude Medical

Prosthetic Valve
Mechanical Prosthesis

Mechanical bileaflet prosthetic valves are used in the aortic position. (A) Represents the surgical view during valve implant; the arrow indicates the cardioplegia cannula in the left coronary ostium. (B) 2D color compare deep TG view assesses paravalvular leaks minimizing the acoustic shadow from the mechanical valve. (D) Leaflet excursion can be appreciated in xPlane ME AV SAX and LAX views. (C) 3D FV of the AVR from ME LAX view is rotated to the surgical orientation (compare with A). Significant echo dropout is present. (E) The FV dataset can be rotated 180° to view the AV prosthesis from the LVOT side.

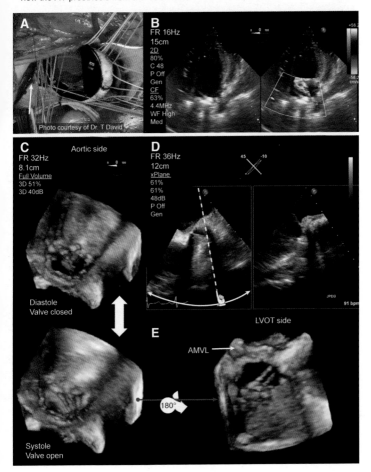

Prosthetic Valve
Mechanical Prosthesis Dehiscence

Patient presents for percutaneous closure of a large paravalvular leak on a mechanical tilting disc (Bjork-Shiley) MVR. (A) 3D Zoom in the surgeon's orientation displays in detail the valve structure and a large posterior gap (arrow). A catheter was positioned (B) over which an Amplatzer® device (C, arrow) was deployed. (D) The color Doppler 3D dataset was imported into QLab (Philips Medical Systems) and the gap measured. Compare (E) the initial leak and (F) after deployment with a smaller residual leak as identified with 3D color Doppler.

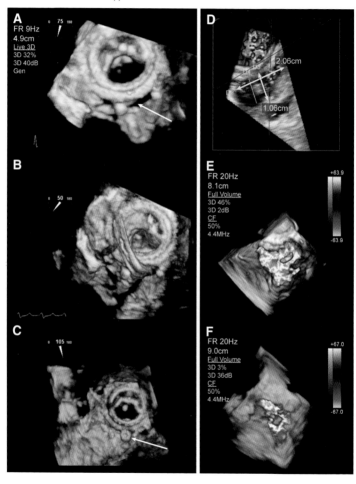

Prosthetic Valve
Prosthesis Thrombosis

Patient with L-TGA and previous mechanical TVR presented for redo surgery with thrombosis of the mechanical prosthesis. An immobile leaflet (arrow) was seen in (A) 2D ME view and confirmed by (B) 2D color Doppler. (C) 3D Zoom en face view of the mechanical prosthesis in the surgical orientation is shown. Lack of one leaflet opening was seen in (E) 3D FV and confirmed with (D) 3D color Doppler.

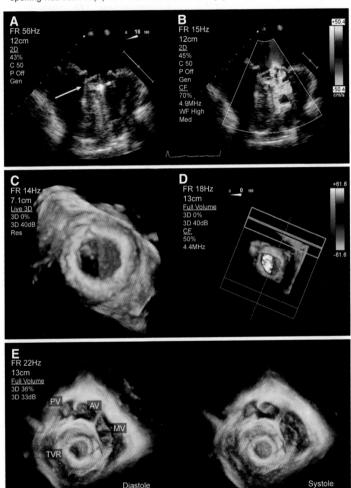

Prosthetic Valve
Bioprosthesis

Stented bioprosthetic valve is comprised of 3 stents supporting 3 leaflets composed of either (A) bovine pericardium or a (B) porcine heterograft. (C) Bioprosthetic MVR shown using (C) 2D and 3D Zoom from the (D) LA side and (E) LV side. This patient had a paravalvular leak shown by arrow (D, E) in 3D TEE and (G) 2D color Doppler. (F) The leak was closed percutaneously using 2 Amplatzer® devices.

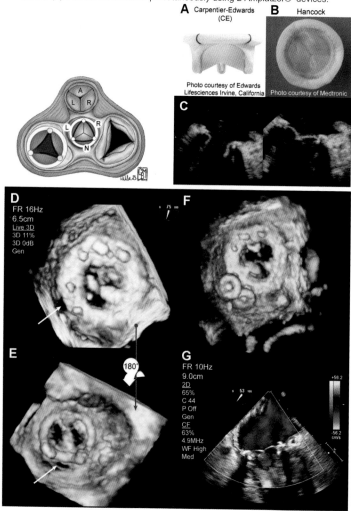

120

Prosthetic Valve
Bioprosthesis

(A) Surgical view of stented AV bioprosthesis after implant. The arrows indicate cardioplegia cannula in the right and left coronary ostia. Deep TG view commonly measures the transvalvular gradient and (B) color compare detects paravalvular leaks during diastole. (D) xPlane ME AV views assess valve stability and leaflet movement simultaneously in SAX and LAX. (C) 3D Zoom from ME AV LAX view is rotated to the surgical orientation (compare with A). 3D color Doppler from ME and TG views can detect paravalvular leaks. (E) 3D color Doppler of AV bioprosthesis with central AI in the surgical orientation from the ME AV LAX view.

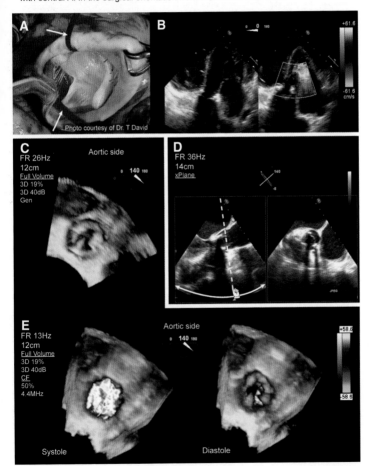

Transcatheter Valve
Native Valve

Assessment of the native aortic valve includes:

- Calcium location (A) 3D Zoom LVOT side, (B) 2D xPlane ME AV LAX, SAX and (C) 3D Zoom aortic side
- (A, B, C) Leaflet mobility in ME AV LAX, SAX
- Annulus measurement (D) 2D ME AV LAX, (E) 2D deep TG LAX
- Color Doppler (F) xPlane ME AV LAX and SAX

Source: Moss RR, et al. JACC Imag 2008;1:15-24.
Zamarano JL, et al. J Am Soc Echocardiogr 2011; 24:937-65.

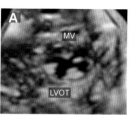

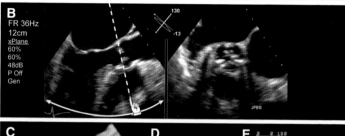

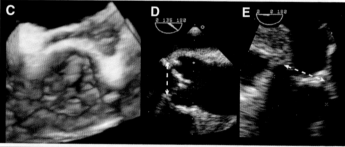

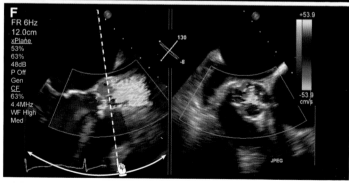

Transcatheter Valve
Edwards Sapien Valve

Annulus Size	Valve Size
18–22 mm	23 mm
21–25 mm	26 mm
24–28 mm	29 mm

Photo of Transcatheter Heart Valve (THV) courtesy
Edwards Lifesciences
Irvine, California

Edwards Sapien THV

The procedure involves placement of a balloon catheter mounted valve, delivered either retrograde through a transfemoral or antegrade transapical LV approach. The native valve is first dilated by balloon valvuloplasty. (A) 3D Live ME AV LAX views from the LVOT shows the catheter wire (arrow) through the stenotic AV and balloon inflation. (B) The catheter mounted percutaneous valve is then positioned across the native AV using fluoroscopy and TEE 3D Live ME AV LAX from LVOT. The balloon is inflated to deploy the valve during a period of rapid ventricular pacing to prevent valve embolization.

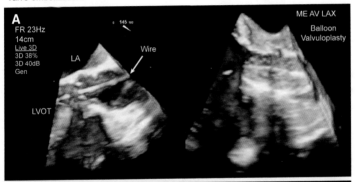

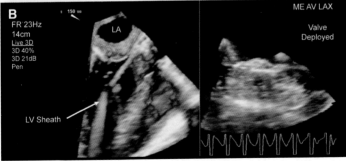

Transcatheter Valve Positioning

Positioning of the Edwards Sapien Transcatheter Heart Valve (THV) before deployment is a key step of this procedure. (A) Correct positioning must take into account a 2–3 mm forward displacement of the catheter mounted valve during deployment using either the transapical or transfemoral approach. (B) Accurate positioning requires valve equator alignment slightly below the native AV annulus (red arrow), 2D ME AV LAX transapical approach. (C) TEE is integrated with fluoroscopy. Examples in 2D ME AV LAX views of THV malpositioning that is (D) too ventricular or (E) too aortic.

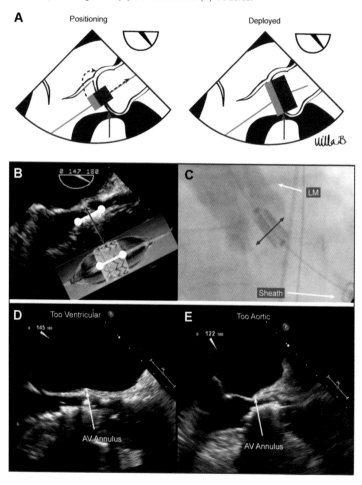

124

Transcatheter Valve
Post-deployment Assessment

Post-deployment assessment uses different modalities to evaluate valve position and stability and assess LV function and coronary blood flow (fluoroscopy). (A) 2D ME AV SAX and (B) 2D ME AV LAX views are shown during diastole with the valve closed. 3D Zoom images from the (C) ascending aortic side during diastole and systole or (D) from LVOT side. (E) Fluoroscopy of the deployed valve also assesses valve function and position.

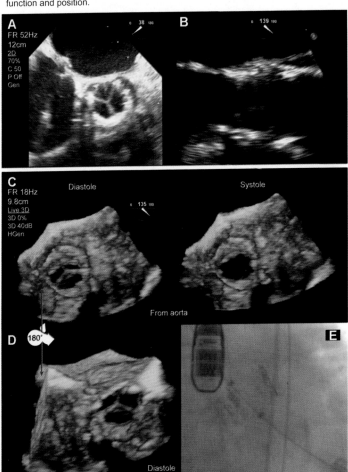

Transcatheter Valve Complications

Common complications during percutaneous AV deployment include (A) catheter malposition (arrow) shown here through the mitral valve in 2D ME AV LAX and (B) paravalvular leaks. The same paravalvular leak (arrow) is shown by color Doppler (B) 2D ME AV LAX, (C) zoomed 2D deep TG, (D) 2D ME AV SAX, (E) 3D deep TG and (F) 3D deep TG rotated to view en face from the LVOT. This is a mild leak but a severe paravalvular leak may require additional balloon dilatation.

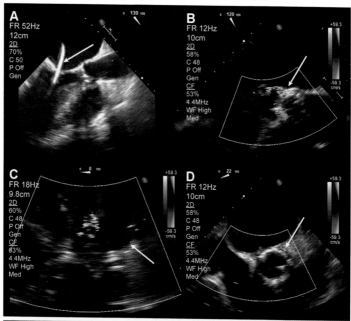

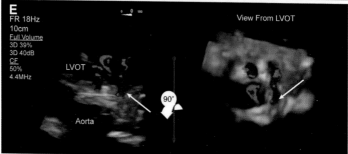

Transcatheter Valve Complications

Rare severe perioperative complications include:

- Systemic valve embolization to mid-aortic arch that occurred during valve deployment as seen with (A) fluoroscopy and (B) 2D UE Aortic Arch LAX view.
- Pericardial effusion and tamponade are likely from ventricular perforation during catheter positioning as seen in (C) 2D TG mid SAX view.
- Acute left main (LM) coronary occlusion (arrow) from displaced calcium following balloon valvuloplasty (D) diagnosed with angiography.
- Early postoperative LV apical pseudoaneurysm (arrow) following a transapical approach in 2D (E) ME 4C and (F) ME 4C color Doppler views.

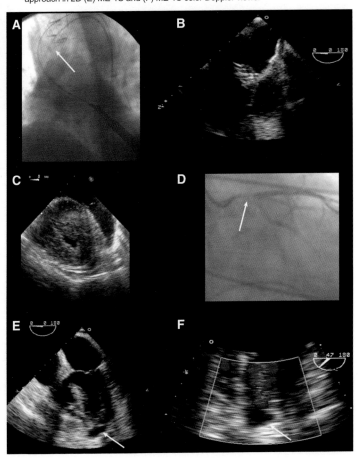

Transcatheter Valve
CoreValve

The Medtronic CoreValve is a bioprosthetic valve encased in a self-expandable nitinol stent. The CoreValve is internally contained and self-deploys during catheter withdrawal. (A) The valve is implanted using a transfemoral approach in patients with symptomatic severe AS, deemed too high a risk for conventional surgery. Baseline TEE is necessary to confirm AV annular measurements and assess other valves and ventricular function. (B) After balloon valvuloplasty the stent is deployed over the coronary ostia without causing significant blood flow obstruction (C). (D) Stent positioning and deployment are done under fluoroscopic guidance alone.

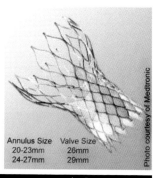

Annulus Size	Valve Size
20-23mm	26mm
24-27mm	29mm

Photo courtesy of Medtronic

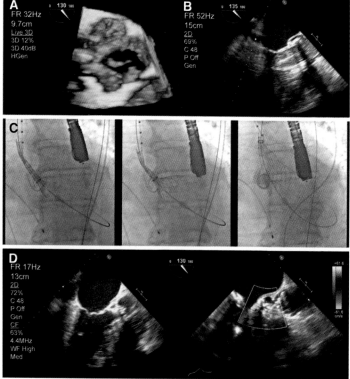

Transcatheter Valve
CoreValve

Post-deployment TEE aims to assess LV, MV, and prosthetic AV function and rule out the presence of paravalvular leaks. (A) 3D Zoom provides consistent en face views of the AV. (B) Fluoroscopy and xPlane allows quick assessment of the deployed prosthesis in (C) 2D and (D) with color. Color Doppler (E) ME LAX and (F) deep TG views are commonly used to assess paravalvular leaks. This patient had a mild posterior paravalvular leak (arrow) better demonstrated in the modified TG view. 3D color Doppler may be a valuable aid in localizing paravalvular leaks.

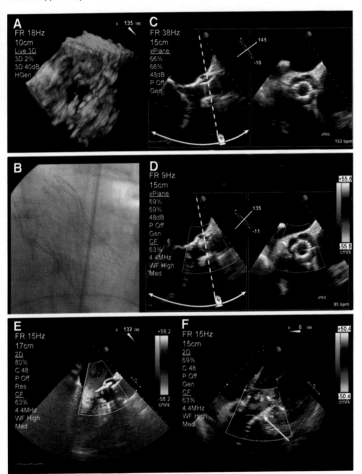

5

Left and Right Ventricles 3D Imaging

A. Vegas et al., *Real-Time Three-Dimensional Transesophageal* 131
Echocardiography, DOI 10.1007/978-1-4614-0665-5_5,
© Springer Science+Business Media, LLC 2012

Left Ventricle
Measurements

LV Size (diastole) Adapted from Lang et al. J Amer Soc Echocardio 2005;18:1440-63.	Reference Range	Mild Abnormal	Moderate Abnormal	Severe Abnormal
LV diastolic diameter (LVDd), cm	M 3.9–5.3 F 4.2–5.9	M 6.0–6.3 F 5.4–5.7	M 6.4–6.8 F 5.8–6.1	M ≥ 6.9 F ≥ 6.2
LV diastolic volume, ml	M 67–155 F 56–104	M 156–178 F 105–117	M 179–201 F 118–130	M ≥ 201 F ≥ 131
Fractional shortening, %	M 25–43 F 27–45	M 20–24 F 22–26	M15–19 F 11–12	M ≤ 14 F ≤ 16
Ejection fraction, %	≥ 55	45–54	30–44	< 30
LV mass index, g/m²	M 49–115 F 43–95	M 116–131 F 96–108	M 132–148 F 109–121	≥ 149 > 122
Relative wall thickness, cm	M 0.24–0.42 F 0.22–0.42	M 0.43–0.46 F 0.43–0.47	M 0.47–0.51 F 0.48–0.52	≥ 0.52 ≥ 0.53

LV mass = $0.8 \times \{1.04[(\text{LVID} + \text{PWT} + \text{SWT})^3 - (\text{LVID})^3]\} + 0.6$ g
LV mass index = LV mass/BSA
Relative wall thickness = $(2 \times \text{PWT})/\text{LVID}$

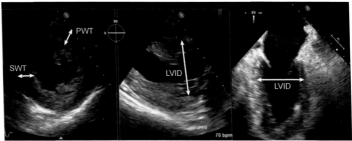

LV stroke volume by Doppler
Stroke volume (SV) = $\pi\,(D/2)^2$ X VTI
- LVOT cross-sectional area (measure diameter [D] in 2D ME AV LAX view)
- Velocity time integral (VTI) of flow at LVOT level (measure in 2D TG LAX view)
  - Avoids LV geometric assumptions
  - Normal SV: 55 ± 10 (36–82) cc/m²

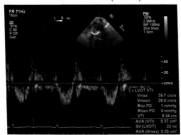 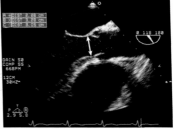

Left Ventricle
2D Assessment

Quantitative assessment of LV systolic function includes estimates of stroke volume (SV) and ejection fraction (EF) by M-mode (FS), 2D (FAC and Simpson's), and Doppler echocardiography. Accurate volume calculations using TEE are difficult as assumptions are made about symmetric LV shape and uniform global function. Load conditions may affect indices of systolic function. Technical limitations include inadequate endocardial border definition and avoidance of LV foreshortening. 3D TEE overcomes some of these limitations (see pgs. 136,139).

Fractional Shortening (FS)

Linear measurement
In TG mid SAX view, measure the end-diastolic (LVIDd) and end-systolic (LVIDs) diameters using M-mode.
FS poorly reflects overall LV function as it assesses only mid- or basal segments.
It assumes the LV has an ellipsoid shape with a 2:1 long axis/short axis ratio.

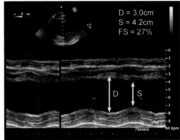

$$FS\ (\%) = \frac{LVID_d - LVID_s}{LVID_d} \times 100\%$$

Normal FS > 30%

Fractional Area Change (FAC)

Area measurement
In TG mid SAX view, planimeter the endocardial border (exclude papillary muscles) to obtain LV end-diastolic area (LVEDA) and end-systolic area (LVESA). It assumes normal global function with no wall motion abnormalities.

LVEDA 9.79 cm²   LVESA 5.79cm²

$$FAC\ (\%) = \frac{LVEDA - LVESA}{LVEDA} \times 100\%$$

Normal FAC 45–80%

Modified Simpson's Method
Method of Discs

Volume measurement
Trace endocardial border, during ES, ED in ME 4C, ME 2C begin and end at the MV annulus. The ventricle is divided into discs. The volume of each disc is automatically calculated for the 20 discs and summed giving the EDV and ESV.

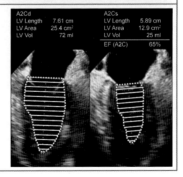

A2Cd		A2Cs	
LV Length	7.61 cm	LV Length	5.89 cm
LV Area	25.4 cm²	LV Area	12.9 cm²
LV Vol	72 ml	LV Vol	25 ml
		EF (A2C)	65%

Stroke Volume (SV) = EDV – ESV
Ejection Fraction (EF %) = SV / EDV

Normal SV = 55 ± 10 (36–82) cc/m²

Left Ventricle
xPlane

xPlane mode displays two 2D planes simultaneously (see pg. 5). The left display is the base TEE plane. The right display is the second plane which by default is at 90°, bisecting the base plane (dotted line). This mode is convenient to assess multiple LV wall segments (ASE 17 segment model) in a single display. (A) ME 4C and 2C views image four LV walls (13 segments) at the same time. The right plane can be tilted (−5°) to cut through the true LV apex. (B) TG mid SAX and TG 2C views assess 10 segments. All segments are evaluated for motion and thickening.

Wall Score		Wall Motion	% Radius Change	Wall Thickening	
1	Normal	Inward	> 30%	+++	30–50%
2	Mild	Inward	10–30%	++	30–50%
3	Severe	Inward	< 10%	+	< 30%
4	Akinesis	None	None	0	< 10%
5	Dyskinesis	Outward	None	0	None

Wall Motion Score Index (WMSI) = sum of wall motion scores / number of visualized segments
Normal WMSI = 1, WMSI > 1.7 indicates perfusion defect > 20%

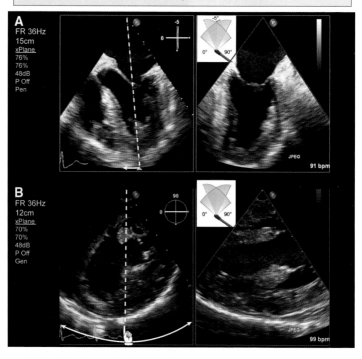

134

Left Ventricle
LV 3D Full Volume

3D LV quantification uses FV datasets that include the entire LV cavity with an adequate frame rate to analyze LV motion. (A) FV acquisition starts with a biplane preview of optimized 2D ME 4C and 2C views. Choose a FV acquisition option (4 or 7 beats) and line density that includes the entire LV (see pg. 12). Avoid any probe or patient movement and ECG artifacts during FV acquisition to prevent stitch artifacts. (B,C) Rotate the entire FV 3D dataset downward to show the MV from the LA and check for stitch artifacts (see pg. 21). Discard the 3D dataset if stitch artifacts are present. (D) The entire LV FV 3D dataset is 50% cropped to show the LV cavity interior but adds little to LV function assessment. Further quantification of LV function requires exporting the FV 3D dataset to analytical software.

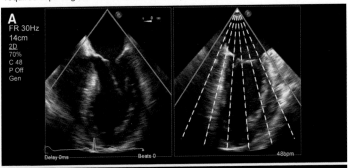

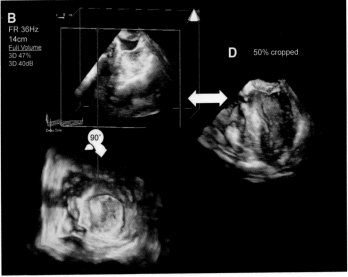

Left Ventricle
3D Guided Biplane Method

The LV FV dataset is exported for analysis into a quantification software (3DQ QLab, Philips Medical Systems). LV volumes can be measured with RT 3D TEE using 2 methods: 3D-guided biplanes or direct volumetric analysis.
(A) The FV dataset is displayed on three MPRs (multiplanar reconstructions **G**reen, **R**ed, **B**lue). (B) To use the 3D guided biplane method of discs for a TEE LV 3D dataset, the red and green planes are adjusted to cut the LV along its long axis at the true apex. Ideal (C) ME 4C and (D) ME 2C views are created that minimize LV foreshortening. The endocardium and the epicardium are traced in diastole and systole. Automatic measurements and calculations include: Stroke Volume, Ejection Fraction, End Diastolic and End Systolic volumes, and LV mass.

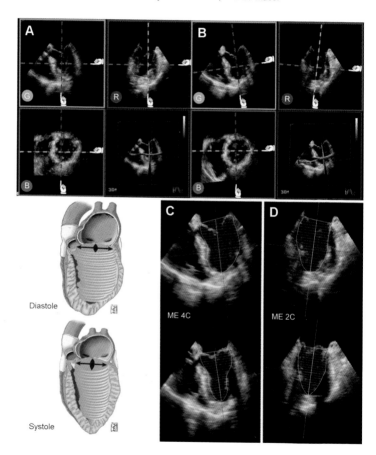

Diastole

Systole

ME 4C

ME 2C

Left Ventricle
i-slice

The i-slice view shows unforeshortened dynamic sagittal (SAX) cuts through different LV levels from apex to base. Endocardial motion can be viewed in 16, 9, or 4 simultaneous clips. This method qualitatively and quantitatively assesses all LV wall segments. Careful positioning of the MPRs (**R**ed, **G**reen, **B**lue) are required to avoid foreshortening the LV and accurately locate the i-slice planes perpendicular to the LV long axis.

1. The red and green MPRs are first positioned (hand icons) in the mid LV cavity through the true LV apex.
2. The blue MPR is then adjusted perpendicular to red and green lines in the green and red panels, respectively. The LV SAX view is displayed in the blue panel.

At any time predetermined 4, 9, or 16 planes view can be chosen increasing the density of the 2D planes in one view. Plane 1 cuts through the more basal LV portion, and plane 16 through the apical region.

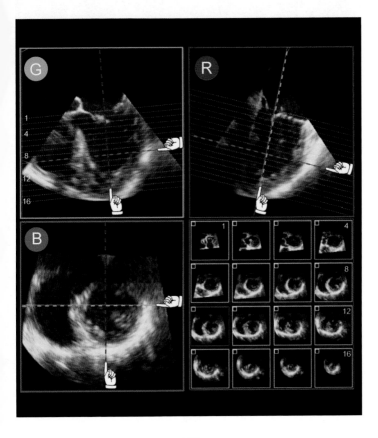

Left Ventricle
LV model

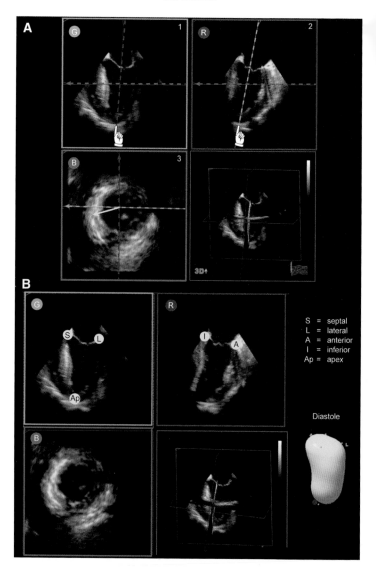

S = septal
L = lateral
A = anterior
I = inferior
Ap = apex

Diastole

138

Left Ventricle
3D Global Function

To generate a dynamic LV endocardial cast, the 3D FV dataset is imported into the analytical software (3DQA, QLab, Philips Medical Systems) and analyzed as follows:
1. Identify the end-diastolic frame (A1)
2. Align MPR axis (red and green lines) through LV apex in 2C and 4C views (A1,A2)
3. Identify middle of IVS in blue panel using yellow arrow (A3)
4. Add reference points to the LV walls (4C S+L, 2C I+A) and apex (B)
5. Repeat procedure for end-systolic frame

(A) Following sequence analysis, a 3D endocardial shell is surface rendered with a graph of global LV volume over time for each frame of the cardiac loop. (B) The end-diastolic volume (EDV) and end-systolic volume (ESV) are measured and stroke volume (SV) and ejection fraction (EF) are automatically calculated and shown. The maximum (blue) and minimum (red) ventricular volumes are shown by the dots. The EDV and ESV measured by this direct volume technique differs from the single frame method of discs (see pg. 136). The latter technique slightly overestimates ventricular volumes but is currently the ASE preferred method for LV volume assessment.

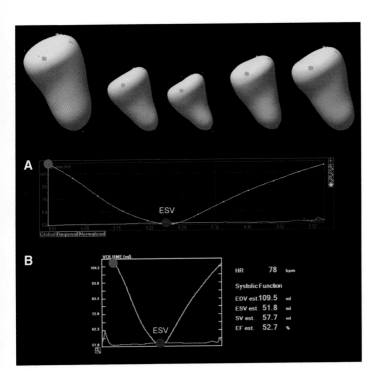

Left Ventricle
Segmental Model

AHA 17 Segment LV Model		
Basal Segments	**Mid Segments**	**Apical Segments**
1. Basal anterior	7. Mid anterior	13. Apical anterior
2. Basal antero-septal	8. Mid antero-septal	14. Apical septal
3. Basal infero-septal	9. Mid infero-septal	15. Apical inferior
4. Basal inferior	10. Mid inferior	16. Apical lateral
5. Basal infero-lateral	11. Mid infero-lateral	17. Apex
6. Basal antero-lateral	12. Mid antero-lateral	

The 17 segment LV model was created in 2002 by the AHA as a consensus guide-line to describe LV segmental anatomy for all cardiac imaging modalities. It is used to describe LV regional wall motion and includes a true apical segment devoid of cavity.
Source: Cerqueira M, et al. Circulation 2002;105:539-42

All LV segments are imaged using both the TG SAX and ME views.

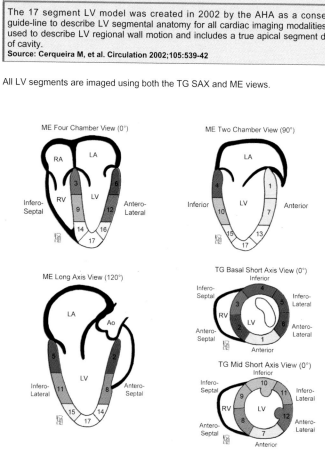

Left Ventricle
Segmental Analysis

The dynamic LV cast can be (A) automatically divided into 17 wedges that correspond to (B) the AHA 17 segment LV model in TTE orientation. 3D TEE assessment of regional LV wall motion is based on a change in LV chamber volume over time from altered segmental myocardial contractility. Unlike standard 2D TEE, there is no direct measurement of myocardial thickening or displacement of individual segments. The change in volume of each wedge is displayed as (C) an absolute volume or (D) as a percentage of the end-diastolic volume of each wedge. The sum of the absolute values is the stroke volume. A zero value means the LV segment is akinetic. The red triangles indicate the time to minimal systolic volume (TMSV) of each wedge and their distribution allows visualization of overall ventricular synchronicity.

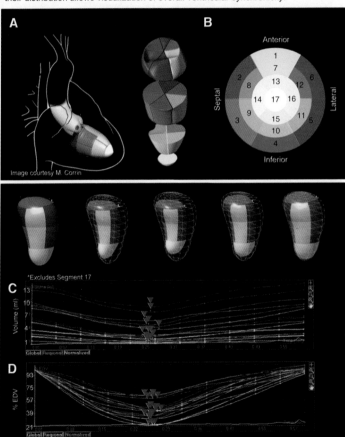

Left Ventricle
Segmental Analysis

(A) At any time during segmental analysis the cursor (hand icon) can be moved over a single trace and it will highlight the corresponding wedge on the 3D model and the 17 segment bull's eye. This highlighted trace corresponds to LV segment 1 (basal anterior) with time and volume as indicated.

Parametric imaging displays as bull's eye diagrams of ASE 17 segment LV model in TTE orientation with analysis of (B) segmental timing and (C) excursion. (B) Normal timing is shown in green, premature contraction as blue, and delayed contraction as red. (C) Inward movement (normal excursion) is displayed as blue, no movement (akinesis) is black and outward movement (dyskinesis) as red.

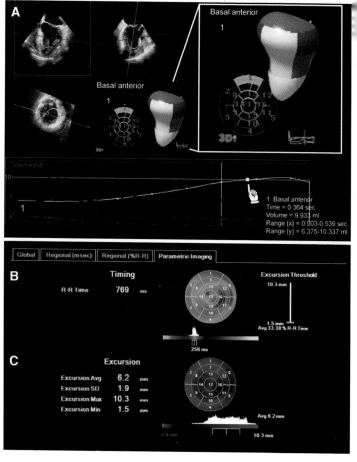

Left Ventricle
Regional Wall Motion

LV wall motion abnormalities can be promptly recognized by assessing the end-systolic frame in relation to the overlying end-diastolic reference mesh. The bull's eye diagram confirms the diagnosis and provides measurements of global LV excursion (average, min, max and SD). (A) Normal LV function in a patient undergoing mitral valve repair. (B) Antero-septal akinesis from an anterior MI (arrow) after a Bentall procedure. (C) Apical aneurysm and basal antero-lateral akinesis (arrow) scheduled for aortic valve replacement for aortic stenosis.

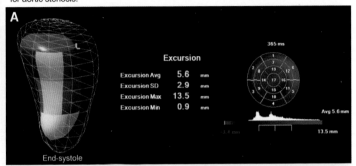

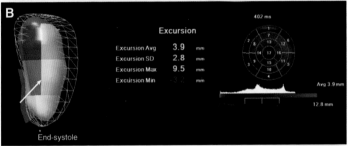

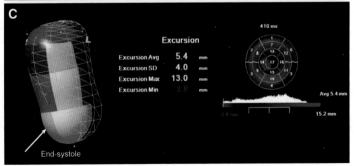

Left Ventricle
Dysynchrony

In a normal heart, ventricular activation spreads through the AV node, His bundle, left and right bundles and the Purkinje system. Normal contraction is impaired with bundle branch block (BBB) and or systolic dysfunction resulting in intraventricular or interventricular dysynchrony. Tissue Doppler Imaging (TDI) is a common technique to assess this using peak systolic velocity of different LV segments.

Using off-line analysis, timing from the start of the QRS to peak systolic contraction is obtained for different LV segments using the ME 4C, 2C and LAX views.

(A) Normal intraventricular synchrony of 50 msec is shown between antero-septal (green) and infero-lateral (yellow) walls. Intraventricular dysynchrony is suggested by:

- Difference > 60 msec between septum and lateral wall
- Maximal difference > 60 msec between any 2 segments
- Standard deviation > 32 msec between 16 segments

(B) Interventricular dysynchrony is the difference between the aortic ejection time (AET, start of the QRS to the start of ejection through the aortic annulus) and (C) pulmonary ejection time (PET, start of the QRS to the start of ejection through the pulmonic valve). The normal difference in timing is < 40 ms.

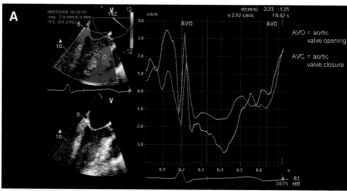

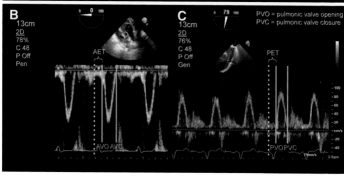

144

Left Ventricle
Dysynchrony

3D echocardiography can also assess intraventricular dysynchrony. Systolic dysynchrony index (SDI) is defined as the standard deviation of the time taken to reach minimum systolic volume (TMSV) for each segment as a percentage of the cardiac cycle (%R-R). For normal subjects, the mean SDI (16 segment model) is 3.5% ± 1.8%. The cardiac apex (segment 17) is excluded from analysis despite being displayed on the parametric bull's eye.

(A) Delayed septal contraction without wall motion abnormalities is shown. These figures are generated from segmental analysis of the 3D LV model showing composite report pages (A1) regional TMSV in msec, (A2) regional TMSV as %R-R, (B,C) parametric or polar display, and (D) volume over time plot. It is reported for 16 (apical cap excluded), 12 (basal + mid), and 6 (basal) segments as a standard deviation (SD) or averaged difference (Diff). The 2 polar graphs display timing (C) and excursion (B) for each of the 17 ASE segments. Normal timing is shown in green, premature contraction as blue and delayed contraction as red. (D) When LV dysynchrony is present, the minimum systolic volume of each wedge (triangles) is scattered over time.

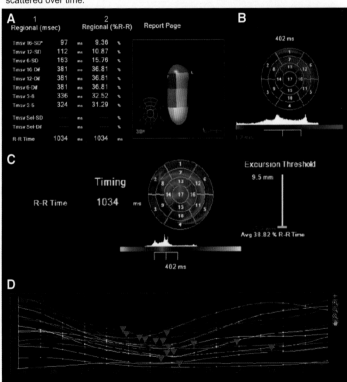

Left Ventricle
Strain

Myocardial strain is the deformation of the cardiac muscle and has been used to quantify myocardial systolic function. It is calculated as percent or fractional change in dimension. The strain measure is named Langrangian strain.

$$\text{Strain (e)} = (L - L_0) / L$$

Three types of strain can be measured: circumferential, radial (TG SAX), and longitudinal (ME 4C, 3C, and 2C). By convention, lengthening and thickening are given positive values, whereas shortening and thinning are assigned negative values. Strain values can be obtained off-line either using 2D Tissue Doppler Imaging (TDI) or speckle tracking imaging. The major advantage of speckle-tracking imaging is that it is independent of angle/cardiac translation. (A) TDI with curved M-Mode of the lateral LV wall from the ME 4C view. Sample points are set on the lateral LV wall and the velocities are plotted over time on the right. (B) Radial strain is assessed from a TG SAX view.

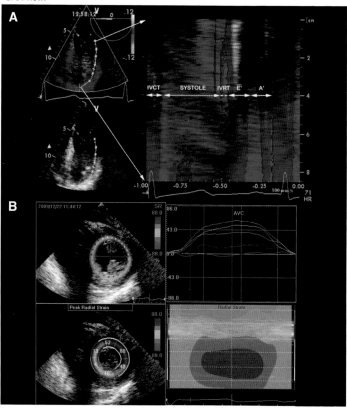

146

Left Ventricle
Strain

Speckle tracking imaging showing longitudinal strain of LV in ME 4C (A) and 2C (B) TEE views. Normal strain pattern shows little deviation of each color coded segments. (A) Decreased longitudinal strain of akinetic basal (1)(red) and hypokinetic mid (−4)(blue) antero-lateral segments. (B) Decreased longitudinal strain (−3)(red) of hypokinetic basal anterior segment.

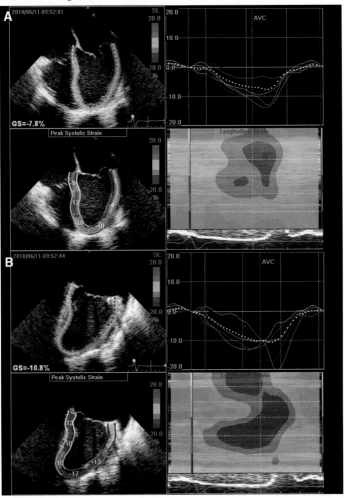

Right Ventricle
Dimensions

RV size (diastole) Adapted from Lang et al. J. Amer Soc Echocardiogr 2005;18:1440-63.	Reference Range	Mild Abnormal	Moderate Abnormal	Severe Abnormal
RV dimensions (Fig. A)				
Basal RV diameter (RVD1), cm	2.0–2.8	2.9–3.3	3.4–3.8	**≥ 3.9**
Mid-RV diameter (RVD2), cm	2.7–3.3	3.4–3.7	3.8–4.1	**≥ 4.2**
Base-to-apex length (RVD3), cm	7.1–7.9	8.0–8.5	8.6–9.1	**≥ 9.2**
RV diastolic area, cm²	11–28	29–32	33–37	**≥ 38**
RV systolic area, cm²	7.5–16	17–19	20–22	**≥ 23**
RV fractional area change, %	32–60	25–31	18–24	**≥ 17**
RVOT diameters (Fig. B)				
Below aortic valve (RVOT1), cm	2.5–2.9	3.0–3.2	3.3–3.5	**≥ 3.6**
Below pulmonic valve (RVOT2), cm	1.7–2.3	2.4–2.7	2.8–3.1	**≥ 3.2**

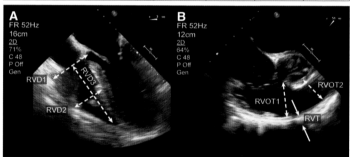

Normal RV wall thickness (RVT) < 5 mm
    RV hypertrophy (RVH) > 7 mm, occurs with pressure overload
Normal RV area < 0.6 LV area,
Normal RV length < 0.6 LV length

Qualitative RV function assessment includes RV free wall motion using Live 3D (A) ME 4C, (B) TG RV SAX, (C) TG RV inflow and Full Volume (D) RVOT view.

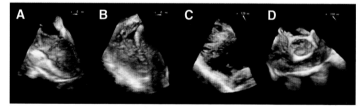

Right Ventricle
Function

Pericardial Septal Motion
Pericardial constraint restricts interventricular septal (IVS) wall motion.
Findings associated with abnormal constraint:
- Reciprocal ventilatory changes in RV and LV size
- Greater respiratory variation during inspiration and expiration in TV + MV inflow
    - Normal spontaneous: TV < 15%, MV < 10%
    - Constrictive pericarditis: TV > 40%, MV > 25%
    - Tamponade: TV > 85%, ↓ MV > 40% with inspiration
IVS is normally convex toward the RV during the entire cardiac cycle.
- RV pathology results in "D-shaped" septum with abnormal (paradoxical) motion, toward the LV during different parts of the cardiac cycle.
- Assess using **Eccentricity Index (EI)**
    - Normal = 1 at EDD and ESD
    - RV volume overload (EDD) EI > 1, ESD=1
    - RV pressure overload (ESD, EDD) EI > 1

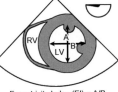

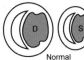

Normal   Volume overload   Pressure overload

Eccentricity Index (EI) = A/B

Right Ventricular Ejection Fraction (RV EF)
RV EF = (RV EDV – RV ESV) / RV EDV
- Load dependent, prognostic value
- Use Simpson's rule or area length method
- Normal value 45–68%

Right Ventricular Fractional Area Change (RV FAC)
RV FAC = (RV EDA - RV ESA) / RV EDA
- Trace RV areas in systole and diastole
- Correlates with RV EF if no regional dysfunction
- Normal 32–60%, mild 25–31%, mod 18–24%, severe < 17%

TAPSE: 20-25mm   ESA

Tricuspid Annular Plane Systolic Excursion (TAPSE)
- Longitudinal motion of lateral TV annulus to cardiac apex
- Measure shortening using M-mode in 4C
- Normal 20–30 mm, impaired systolic motion < 16 mm

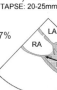

EDA

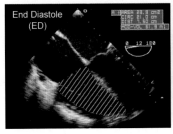

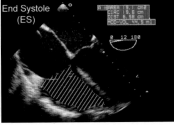

Right Ventricle
TV Annular Velocity

(A) In a minority of patients, a modified deep TG RV view can be obtained by rotating the probe to the right. It allows good ultrasound beam alignment with TV annulus movement. (B) Similar to TTE, the TV annular displacement can be displayed using M-mode and the systolic excursion measured.

(C) TV systolic displacement can also be measured using Tissue Doppler imaging (TDI) from a modified TG RV inflow view (120–130°). Typical TDI trace of TV annular velocity (TAV) consists of 4 waves:

- 2 systolic: isovolumetric contraction (IVC) and systolic (S)
- 2 diastolic: early filling (E) and atrial contraction (A)

IVC and S peak velocities and IVC slope have correlated to RV systolic function.

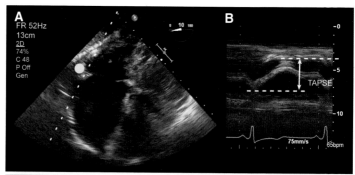

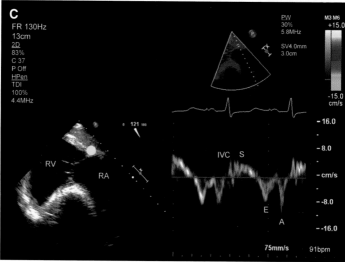

150

Right Ventricle
RV Strain

RV function can be assessed using 2D strain from a modified ME 4C view. The view is obtained by rotating the probe to the right to center the RV on the screen. A 2D loop is obtained at a FR > 40 Hz with the best possible RV free wall endocardial and epicardial definition. Narrowing the sector size helps to increase the FR. The analysis is performed off-line using a speckle tracking system. (A) Most quantification software does not have a specific package for RV strain analysis; thus, the ME 2C view LV settings are normally used. The analysis includes the RV free wall and IVS strain. (B) Average strain can be measured for the RV free wall alone by excluding the trace relative to the IVS. This technique correlates well with TDI as it is angle independent and uses a view that is frequently obtained.

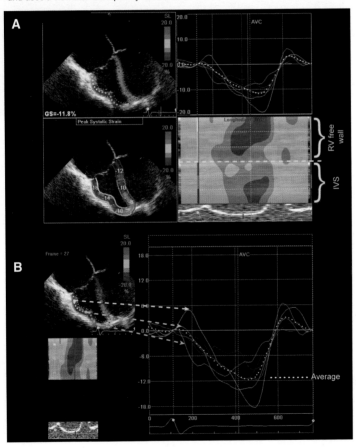

Right Ventricle
xPlane

xPlane mode allows the simultaneous display of two 2D views (see pg. 5). In the assessment of RV function from a modified ME 4C view, the TEE probe can be maneuvered to center the RV on the screen. (A) Choosing xPlane mode displays the RV in a modified ME 4C view in the left panel and a modified ME RV inflow-outflow view in the right panel. Moving the secondary scanning plane left and right (cursor line) the RV free wall can be scanned and displayed on the right panel. (B) From a modified TG LV SAX view, turning the probe to the right centers the RV on the screen. xPlane simultaneously displays the RV in SAX and LAX.

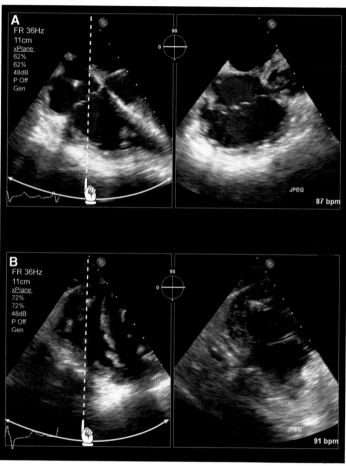

Right Ventricle
i-Slice

RV FV 3D dataset is obtained from a modified ME 4C view rotated to the right to center the RV on the screen. (A) The 3D dataset is exported into a quantification software (3DQA, Philips Medical Systems) for analysis. (B) In diastole the Red plane is positioned in the Green panel, perpendicular to TV annular displacement, and the Blue plane parallel to it. (C) On the end-systolic frame, the first i-slice plane is positioned at the TV annulus level. The i-slice panel density is adjusted to cover the entire RV to the apex. (B) TAPSE can be measured in diastole on the Green panel and corresponds to the distance along the red line between the TV annulus and the first blue plane. (D) Enlarged view of i-slice through SAX of RV from base (1) to apex (9).

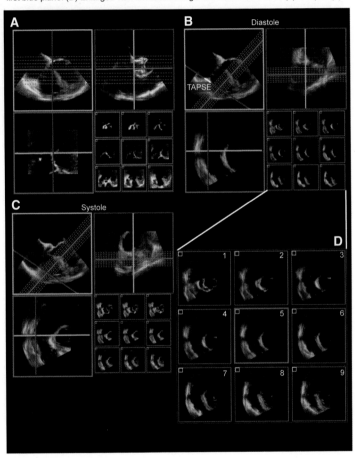

Right Ventricle
RV Model

(A) 3D analysis of the RV cavity can only be performed using special analytical software by TomTec F(4D RV-Function©; TomTec Imaging Systems GmbH, Munich, Germany). (B) Similar to LV quantification, a good quality FV RV 3D dataset is required. TomTec software uses a semi-automated technique. (C) The 3D dataset is displayed on three MPRs. The RV endocardium is manually traced in all MPR planes using (C) the end-diastolic and (D) end-systolic frames. Sequence analysis generates a dynamic model of the RV cavity and displays a plot of the RV volume over time. (E) RV end-diastolic volume (EDV), RV end-systolic volume (ESV), RV ejection fraction (EF) and RV stroke volume (SV) are automatically measured. (F) The 3D model can be rotated and a reference diastolic mesh allows visual estimation of ejection fraction and wall motion abnormalities.

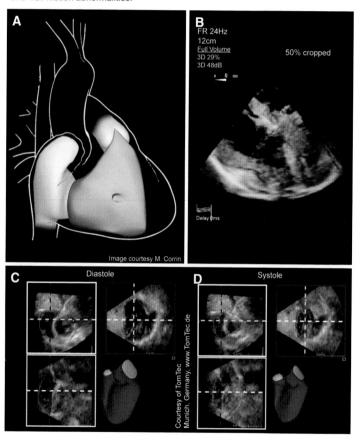

154

Right Ventricle
RV Model

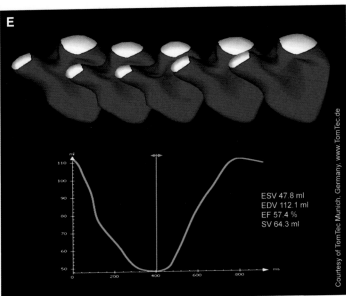

E

ESV 47.8 ml
EDV 112.1 ml
EF 57.4 %
SV 64.3 ml

Courtesy of TomTec Munich, Germany, www.TomTec.de

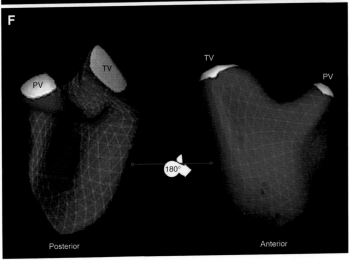

F

PV

TV

180°

TV

PV

Posterior

Anterior

6

Cardiomyopathy Ventricles 3D Imaging

A. Vegas et al., *Real-Time Three-Dimensional Transesophageal Echocardiography*, DOI 10.1007/978-1-4614-0665-5_6, © Springer Science+Business Media, LLC 2012

Hypertrophic Obstructive Cardiomyopathy
Pathophysiology

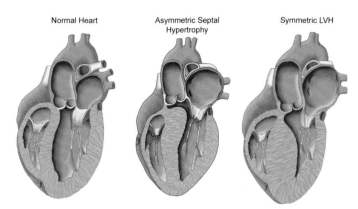

Normal Heart   Asymmetric Septal Hypertrophy   Symmetric LVH

Asymmetric septal hypertrophy has unexplained LV hypertrophy, may have LV obstruction (LVOT or mid-cavitary) and abnormal diastolic function. It is autosomal dominant with variable penetrance, related to abnormalities of the beta myosin heavy chain. Incidence of 1 in 500. Usually asymptomatic though presenting symptoms include LVOT obstruction (syncope, sudden death), myocardial ischemia (angina) and diastolic dysfunction (pulmonary congestion and shortness of breath). Surgery involves a transaortic septal myectomy with an incision parallel to the septum starting below the right coronary cusp and extending to the papillary muscles.

TEE Findings pre CPB
2D Imaging/2D Color Doppler
- LV wall thickness (septal, lateral), symmetric or asymmetrical
    Septal: free wall ratio > 1.3:1, > 15 mm abnormal
- Diameter LVOT, turbulent LVOT flow (color)
- Mitral valve: mitral regurgitation (eccentric posterior directed jet)
    – No intrinsic mitral valve disease
    – Systolic anterior motion (SAM) of the anterior mitral valve leaflet (AMVL)
    – Measure septal contact point
- LA size (LAE) > 40 mm or > 20 cm^2 in ME 4C
- LV and RV systolic function, normal or hyperdynamic
Spectral Doppler
- PW point of peak gradient (check intra-cavitary)
- CW peak and mean LVOT gradient
    – Late peaking systolic flow (dagger shaped)
    – Gradient increases post PVC and amyl nitrate
- MV inflow LV diastolic dysfunction
- Pulmonary vein pattern abnormalities consistent with diastolic dysfunction
3D Imaging/3D Color
- Complete assessment of IVS thickness
- Qualitative assessment of LVOT narrowing
- Spatial representation of regurgitant jets

Hypertrophic Obstructive Cardiomyopathy
Pre-assessment

Typical TEE findings include (A) turbulent flow in the LVOT with posteriorly directed mitral regurgitation in 2D ME AV LAX color Doppler, (B) dagger-shaped CW Doppler trace from deep TG view and (C) systolic anterior motion (SAM) in 2D ME AV LAX view. (D) Turbulent flow across the aortic valve causes fluttering of the AV cusps that can be demonstrated using M-mode in 2D ME AV LAX view.

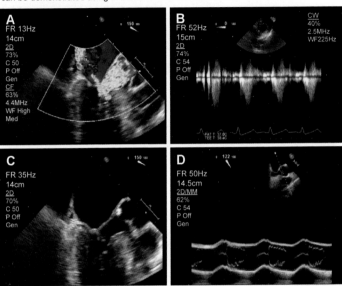

(E) 3D FV ME AV LAX is rotated to the ascending aortic (Asc Ao) orientation to show the IVS protruding into the LVOT through the open AV. (F) 3D Live ME AV LAX view is tilted upward to show SAM (arrow).

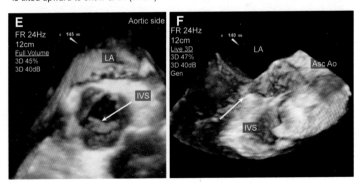

Hypertrophic Obstructive Cardiomyopathy
Systolic Anterior Motion

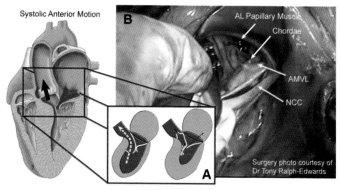

(A) Systolic anterior motion (SAM) of the MV leaflets occurs in early and late systole. As a result of the Venturi effect, the anterior mitral valve leaflet (AMVL) may contact the IVS. Leaflet malcoaptation leads to a posteriorly directed MR jet. (B) The surgeon is pulling the AMVL into the LVOT. SAM is seen in (C) 2D and (D) rotated 3D FV ME AV LAX views to the LVOT side. (E) 2D ME AV LAX color Doppler view demonstrates turbulent flow in the LVOT during systole and a posteriorly directed MR jet. (F) Compare a 3D FV color Doppler AV LAX view rotated to the aortic side to show the turbulent LVOT flow and posteriorly directed MR.

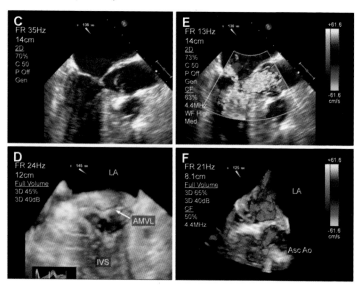

160

Hypertrophic Obstructive Cardiomyopathy
2D vs 3D

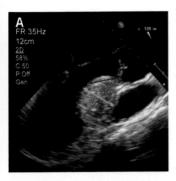

(A) The end-diastolic frame of the 2D TEE ME AV LAX view is used to provide measurements necessary to guide the surgical procedure. The measurements are made on a single slice of the IVS. The challenge is to obtain a plane that is perpendicular to the IVS. An oblique plane overestimates septal thickness.

RCC- SAM septal contact point
Max septal thickness
Min septal thickness
RCC-Min septal thickness

(B) 3D TEE assessment of the LVOT is best done using a 3D FV dataset often acquired from the ME AV LAX view. (C) Using post-acquisition cropping, the arbitrary cropping plane (B, purple) is aligned parallel to the IVS and adjusted to crop through the mid portion of the MV and LV apex. (E) Rotating the cropped 3D image and resetting the standard green cropping plane allow the echocardiographer to obtain an en face view of the LVOT to the AV from the LV. The standard box plane positioned perpendicular to the IVS can be adjusted (B, green) to obtain multiple parallel longitudinal sections of the IVS (D, sample slice). Accurate measurement of the IVS thickness from these 3D views is currently not possible and requires exporting the 3D FV dataset to analytical software.

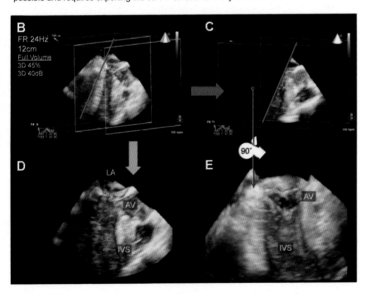

Hypertrophic Obstructive Cardiomyopathy
3D Epiaortic

(A) Epicardial 3D TTE can be performed using a standard X3-1 probe (Philips Medical Systems) covered with a sterile sheath. (B) The epicardial LV LAX (TTE parasternal LAX equivalent) view allows the best image of the IVS. (C,D) xPlane scans the IVS. From a LAX view, the secondary plane is moved along the IVS showing different IVS SAX cuts in the second display. (E) An uncropped TTE FV dataset obtained from the same view can be (F) exported for measurement into the analytical software (Q Lab, Philips Medical Systems). Ongoing studies are assessing the accuracy of IVS measurement using good quality epicardiac views in HOCM patients.

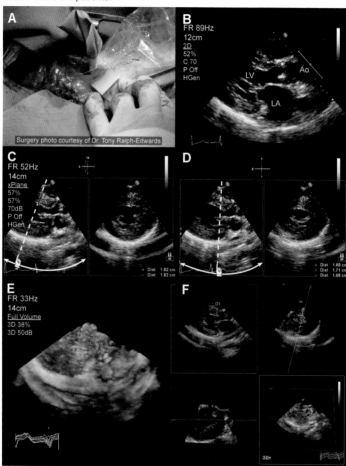

Hypertrophic Obstructive Cardiomyopathy
Quantification

(A) 3DQ, Q Lab software (Philips Medical Systems) allows IVS measurements on multiple planes starting from a FV dataset acquired from a standard ME LAX view. (B,D) Aligning the MPR cuts the IVS in the middle and improves accuracy. (C) A 2D plane can be positioned to cut the LVOT at its narrowest point and provides LVOT cross-sectional area measurements. (E) I slice view shows the IVS on multiple parallel 2D planes and measures it at different levels comparable to an MRI scan.

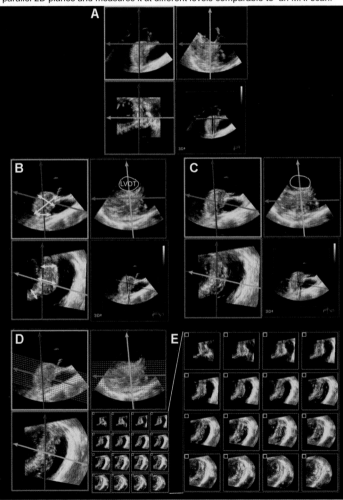

Hypertrophic Obstructive Cardiomyopathy
Surgical Procedure

The IVS is approached through the aortic valve. (A) Following aortotomy, the IVS (arrow) is exposed by retraction of the RCC. (B) 3D FV ME AV LAX dataset seen from the ascending aorta during systole through the aortic valve is very similar to the surgical view. (C) The surgical resection begins 2 cm below the RCC. The depth of the resection is established at the level of the initial cut. The resection must be at least 1 cm below the SAM septal contact point. (D) The resected specimen shows endocardial fibrosis at the SAM septal contact point (arrow). Compare the (E) post-myectomy surgical view with the (A) pre-septal myectomy. (F) Rotated 3D FV ME AV LAX view post-myectomy displays a similar view from the aorta.

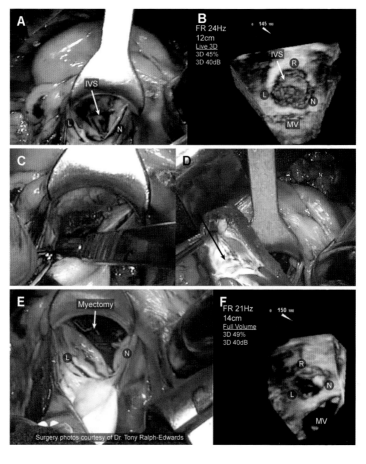

Hypertrophic Obstructive Cardiomyopathy
Post-assessment

TEE Findings post CPB
2D Imaging/Color Doppler
- Measures residual septal thickness
- SAM and residual MR with adequate ventricular filling and blood pressure
- LV and RV systolic function (LAD branches)
- No turbulent (laminar) systolic LVOT flow
- MR from intrinsic valve disease
- R/O VSD (< 3mm IVS), high velocity L to R flow in systole and diastole
- Septal perforator flow in diastole from LV

Spectral Doppler
- CW peak LVOT gradients (post-premature ventricular contraction)
- Mid-ventricular cavitary obstruction
- MV inflow diastolic function
- Pulmonary vein flow

A patient after successful septal myectomy. (A) 2D ME AV LAX color Doppler demonstrates flow acceleration in LVOT. (B) 2D TG LAX CW Doppler measures normal gradient across the LVOT and AV. 3D FV ME AV LAX view in (C) sagittal and (D) rotated to the LVOT side clearly demonstrates the site of myectomy.

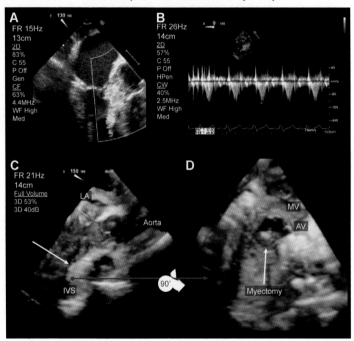

Cardiomyopathy
Subaortic Membrane

Patient with (A) subaortic membrane (arrow) and narrow LVOT shows (B) turbulent flow in 2D ME AV LAX color Doppler views. (C) 3D FV dataset of the LVOT and AV is imported into the quantification software (3DQA, Q Lab, Philips Medical Systems) for measurements. The LVOT cross-sectional area at the level of the membrane is measured at 1.6 cm². (D) 3D color Doppler of the LVOT confirms turbulent flow distal to the membrane. The subaortic membrane can also be appreciated in the 3D FV rotated to the (E) LVOT side and (F) AV in the surgical orientation.

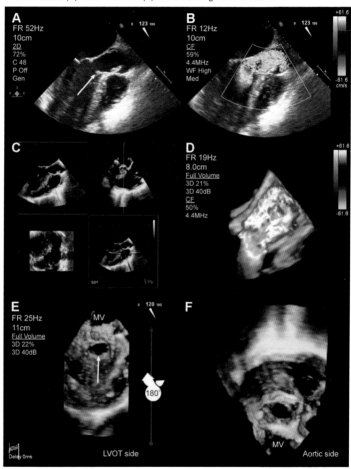

Cardiomyopathy
Subaortic Membrane

(A) Surgery consisted of resection of the fibrous subaortic membrane. The LVOT is free of turbulent flow using (B) 2D and (D) 3D color Doppler. (C) The LVOT cross-sectional area at the level of the previous membrane is now 2.64 cm^2. 3D FV assesses the relieved obstruction (arrow) when viewed from the (E) LVOT side and (F) AV in the surgical orientation compared with the unresected images.

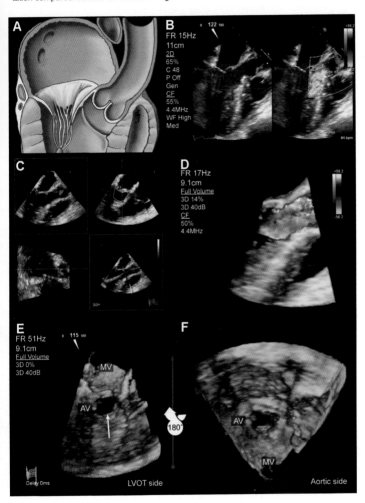

Cardiomyopathy
Left Ventricular Hypertrophy

A patient with LVH and mid-cavitary LV obstruction. The small LV cavity and massive LV hypertrophy are shown in (A) 2D ME 40°, (C) 3D Live ME mitral commissural and (E) 3D FV TG SAX. Turbulent flow in systole results from MR and mid-cavitary obstruction as seen in (B) 2D ME 4C color (arrow) and (D) 2D TG modified LAX. (F) The enlarged post-resection ventricular cavity is seen in 2D TG modified LAX.

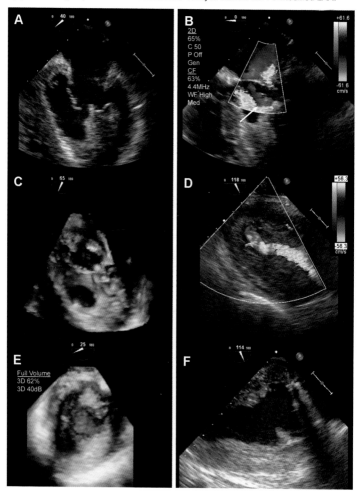

Cardiomyopathy
LV Apical Aneurysm

This is a patient with a large LV apical aneurysm. (A) xPlane mode displays 2 perpendicular ME views of the LV apex. A 3D Full Volume dataset is exported for analysis (3DQA, Q Lab, Philips Medical System). (B) 3D LV reconstruction is performed and parametric displays demonstrate severe apical akinesis (red areas indicate delayed timing and excursion). (C) The end-systolic frame of the LV cast clearly displays an apical aneurysm which can be rotated to the surgical orientation. (D) LV reconstruction after repair displays normal LV geometry. Surgery consisted of (E) resection of LV aneurysm and (F) patch repair.

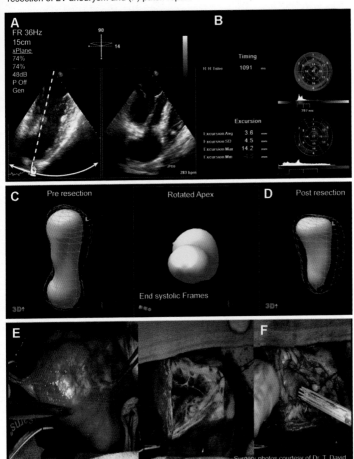

7

Aorta

A. Vegas et al., *Real-Time Three-Dimensional Transesophageal* 171
Echocardiography, DOI 10.1007/978-1-4614-0665-5_7,
© Springer Science+Business Media, LLC 2012

Aorta
Normal Anatomy

Aorta Anatomy

Thoracic aorta is divided into 4 sections:
1. Aortic root: AV to sinotubular junction (STJ)
2. Ascending aorta: STJ to innominate artery
3. Aortic arch: innominate artery to L subclavian artery
4. Descending aorta: distal to L subclavian artery

Aorta wall 3 layers: adventia, media, intima

Size: ascending aorta length: 7–11 cm
      aorta diameter: 35 mm ± 2 mm
      wall thickness 1–2 mm

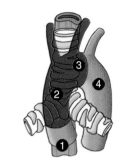

Pathology

- Dilatation (35–50 mm)
- Aneurysm (> 50 mm)
- Dissection (intimal flap)
- Atheromatous disease (plaque, ulceration, hematoma)

Blind spot: region of distal ascending aorta and proximal arch obscured by air-filled trachea and difficult to image with TEE, shown in red above.

3D TEE imaging can be successfully used to view both the thoracic and abdominal aorta. Similar to 2D views, the blind spot limits imaging portions of the aorta.

xPlane (A) 2D and (B) color Doppler display the 2D ME aortic SAX and LAX views of the descending or ascending aorta in 2 side-by-side panels.

Live 3D is obtained from the standard 2D views (C, D) (see pgs. 44–49). It provides real-time information to guide percutaneous techniques, for example, intra-aortic balloon pump insertion (D). Optimize the image by adjusting the gain.

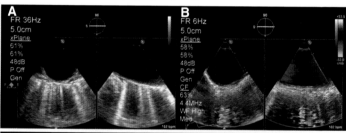

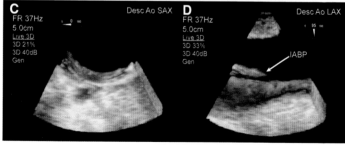

Aorta
3D Assessment

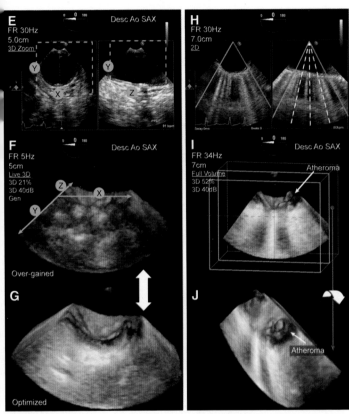

3D Zoom images the aorta with echo dropout in the near field remaining a common problem.
1. Use either a 2D ME Aortic SAX or LAX view to obtain a biplane preview.
2. (E) Position a volume box and adjust x, y, z axes to enclose the entire aorta.
3. (F) Initial Zoom acquisition produces an unrotated over-gained image.
4. (G) Optimize image using reduced gain, smoothing, brightness and magnification.

3D Full Volume (FV) has a larger pyramidal wedge size and higher frame rate which aids assessment of large thin aortic aneurysms and neighboring structures.
1. 3D FV acquisition commences with optimized 2D ME Aortic SAX or LAX view.
2. (H) FV acquisition in a preview image is ECG gated over consecutive heartbeats.
3. (I) Initial FV acquisition is an over-gained image at 50% cropped.
4. (J) Rotate and optimize image using gain, smoothing, brightness and magnification.
5. The crop box can cut the image in any of the 3 axes using 6 planes or free plane.

Aorta
Normal

Image rotation can be performed within any 3D mode using the track ball or Z-rotation function buttons. Rotation provides a circumferential view of the aorta with greater depth appreciation and assessment of complex pathology, patency of intraluminal aortic grafts and detection of atheromatous plaques.

Different parts of the aorta from the aortic root to the descending aorta can be imaged with 3D TEE using both Live 3D and 3D FV. The aortic root can be orientated to show the origins of the coronary arteries. (K) The left main coronary ostia can be seen from the cropped FV ME AV LAX view (arrow). Alternatively an uncropped FV ME AV LAX is rotated to the aortic side to show the (L) left main artery (LMA) and (M) right coronary artery (RCA).

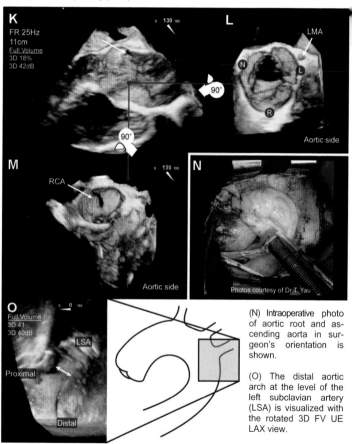

(N) Intraoperative photo of aortic root and ascending aorta in surgeon's orientation is shown.

(O) The distal aortic arch at the level of the left subclavian artery (LSA) is visualized with the rotated 3D FV UE LAX view.

Aorta
Atheroma

Aortic Atheroma
- Location: ascending < arch < descending aorta
- Size
- Consistency: thickened intima, irregular, ± calcium
- Ulcerated plaque ± mobile/sessile components
- Atheroma grading: different grading systems based on echo appearance, though none has proven superior to another

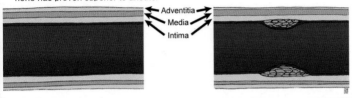

Atheroma Grade (Source: Katz ES, et al. J Am Coll Card 1992; 20:70-77.)
1. Normal aorta
2. Extensive intimal thickening < 3 mm, smooth
3. Protrudes < 5 mm into aortic lumen, irregular, sessile
4. Protrudes > 5 mm into aortic lumen, irregular, sessile (↑ stroke risk)
5. Mobile atheroma of any size (↑ stroke risk)

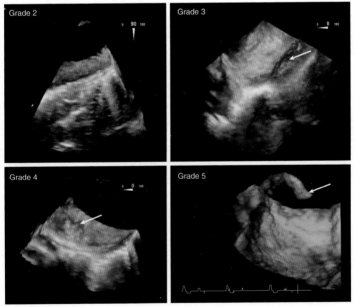

Aorta
Aneurysm

Aortic Aneurysm
- True aneurysm involves dilatation of all wall layers
- Location: ascending, arch, descending aorta
- Size: > 1.5 × normal diameter
- Associated findings (AI, thrombus, atheroma)
- Etiology: atherosclerosis, HBP, AS, Marfan's
- Surgery if sinuses > 40 mm
  - Ascending aorta > 50 mm aortopathy
  - Ascending aorta 55-60 mm no aortopathy

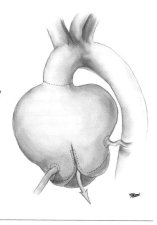

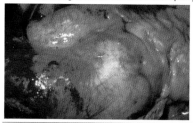

Annuloaortic Ectasia
This condition involves AV annulus dilatation with thinning of the AV cusps and is often associated with Marfan's syndrome. There may be dilatation of the sinuses of valsalva, STJ, ascending aorta, or transverse arch. This patient had a dilatation of the annulus to the ascending aorta with minimal central AI seen with 2D and 3D Live ME AV (A,C) LAX, (B,D) SAX. The patient underwent an AV sparing root replacement ME AV LAX (E) 2D and (F) 3D Live with good AV cusp coaptation.

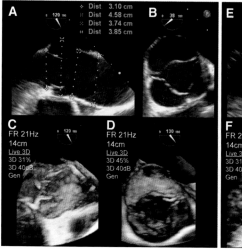

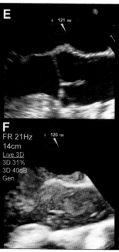

Aorta
Aneurysm

Aortic Root Aneurysm
This patient has a normal sized aortic annulus and AV but dilated aorta extending from the sinuses of Valsalva to mid-ascending aorta as visualized with (A) 2D and (B) over-gained 3D FV acquisition from the ME AV LAX view. An AV sparing root replacement was performed. Good cusp coaptation and view of the coronary ostia are demonstrated with the (C) 2D ME AV LAX and (D) rotated 3D FV AV SAX to show the AV from the ascending aorta.

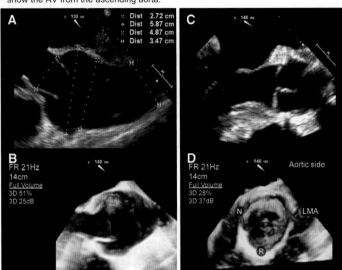

Ascending Aortic Aneurysm
Patient with a calcified bicuspid AV and ascending aortic aneurysm is visualized with (E) 2D and (F) cropped 3D Zoom ME AV LAX views. (G) The uncropped 3D zoom is rotated to view the aneurysm from the aortic side. This patient had a Bentall procedure.

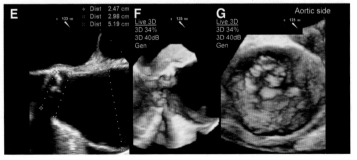

Aorta
Dissection

Tear in intima, blood in media creates a false
lumen with blood flow
Identify intimal flap:
  Discrete sharp edge
  Seen in 2 separate views
  Oscillating, undulating
  Interrupts color flow
  Not outside lumen or cross anatomic planes
Location of entry and exit sites (color Doppler):
  STJ, left subclavian artery
Extent of dissection
True vs. false lumens
Stanford classification
  Type A: ascending aorta
  Type B: descending aorta
Complications:
  Aortic insufficiency (50–70%): quantify, mechanism
  Coronary dissection (10–20%): flap flow
  LV function: global, SWMA
  Pericardial effusion, pleural effusion

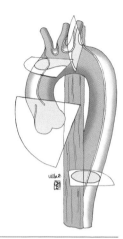

This patient presented with an acute Stanford type A aortic dissection. (A) 2D xPlane
ascending aorta in SAX and LAX, uncropped 3D FV ME AV (B) SAX and (C) LAX
views demonstrate the dissection membrane (green arrow). (D) 3D FV color of ME
AV LAX view shows a perforation (green arrow) within the dissection membrane with
flow between the true lumen (TL) and false lumen (FL).

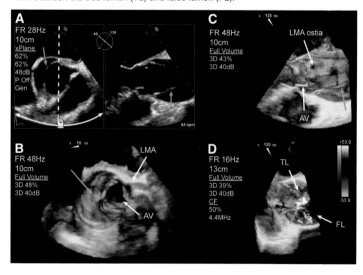

Aorta
Dissection

This patient presented with a dilated ascending aorta and acute type A aortic dissection. The dissection originated at the STJ involving both coronary ostia with moderate AI secondary to prolapse of the dissection membrane as viewed with (A) 2D color Doppler xPlane of the ME AV SAX and LAX views. The membrane (arrow) and large false lumen is demonstrated in the (B) cropped 3D FV ME AV LAX and (C) rotated uncropped LAX view in the surgeon's orientation through the ascending aorta. The dissection extended down to the descending thoracic aorta. False (FL) and true lumens (TL) of the descending aorta are demonstrated in the (D) 2D color xPlane SAX and LAX, (E) 3D Live SAX and (G) rotated 3D Live LAX views.

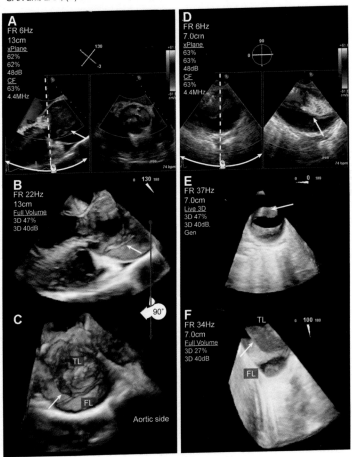

Aorta
Dissection

A patient with Ehler Danlos Syndrome presented for redo surgery with a dilated aortic arch after a previous Bentall procedure. Dilation of the aortic arch and RCA button (arrow) is demonstrated in the (A) 2D, (B) 3D Live UE Aortic Arch SAX and (C) rotated 3D FV LAX views. An associated chronic type B dissection and false aneurysm (arrow) containing thrombus are shown in (D) 2D ME descending aorta LAX, SAX and (E) 3D Zoom LAX views. Replacement of the aortic arch using an elephant trunk technique with reimplantation of both coronary artery buttons was performed. (F) 3D FV UE AA LAX displays the aortic arch graft. (G) The patent elephant trunk within the descending thoracic aorta is visible in the rotated 3D FV ME descending aortic SAX.

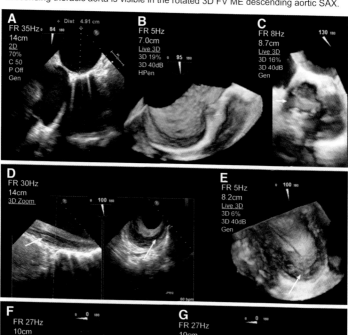

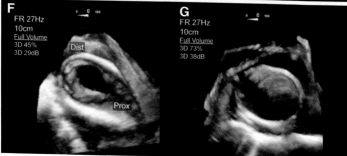

180

Aorta
Thromboembolism

A patient presented with a femoral embolus. (A) Intraoperative TEE for source of embolism showed a mobile structure in the ascending aorta in a 2D color Doppler ME AV LAX view. The patient was found to have a mobile aortic atheroma and underwent resection. (B) The atheroma is shown attached to the ascending aorta intima with an epicardial scan. (C) Unrotated 3D Live AV LAX view and (D) rotated to the ascending aorta in SAX also shows the atheroma. Intraoperative photos of the (E) normal appearing aorta and (F) atheroma are shown during resection.

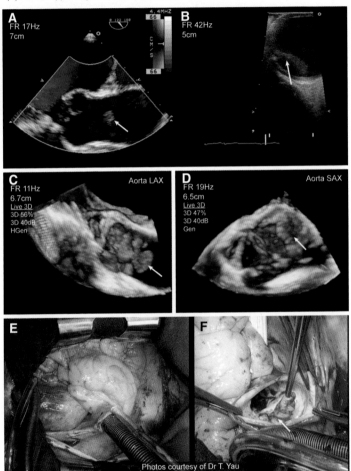

8

Cardiac Masses
3D Imaging

A. Vegas et al., *Real-Time Three-Dimensional Transesophageal* 183
Echocardiography, DOI 10.1007/978-1-4614-0665-5_8,
© Springer Science+Business Media, LLC 2012

Masses
Introduction

Normal Variants

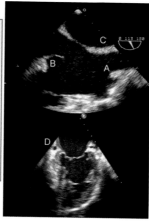

RA
Crista terminalis (A)
Chiari network
Eustachian valve (B)
Pectinate muscles
Thebesian valve
Cannulae
RV
Moderator band
Trabeculations
IAS
Lipomatous hyper-
trophy (C)
IAS aneurysm

LA
Coumadin ridge
Coronary sinus (D)
Pectinate muscles
LV
Aberrant chordae
False tendons
Trabeculations
AV
Nodules of Arantius
Lambl's excrescences
Pericardium
Fat pads
Transverse sinus
Fibrin debris
Cysts
Accessory lobe LAA

Pathological Variants

- Cardiac tumors Primary cardiac tumors are rare (0.03%); majority are metastatic
  - 1° Benign (75%): Myxoma (30%) > lipoma (10%) > papillary fibroelastoma (9%)
    > fibroma (4%)
  - 1° Malignant (25%): Angiosarcoma (9%) > rhabdosarcoma (6%) > mesothelioma
    (2%) > fibrosarcoma (1%)
  - 2° Metastatic: Direct extension: Lung, esophagus, breast
    Intravascular: SVC (lung, thyroid), IVC (renal, hepatoma)
    Hematogenous: Lymphoma, melanoma, leukemia
- Thrombus
- Endocarditis/vegetations

Imaging Masses

3D TEE is an excellent tool for the assessment of cardiac masses and often supplies additional information to the basic 2D examination. The echocardiographic evaluation of masses aims to provide an etiologic differential diagnosis, guide surgical planning, assess tumor resectability, and the need for long-term anticoagulation. The use of 3D TEE ventures further to achieve these goals with greater appreciation of tumor size, location, mobility, attachment sites, surface appearance, embolic potential, cavity obstruction, infiltration of neighboring structures, and presence of associated thrombi and vegetations. This section will focus on imaging a variety of pathological intracardiac masses.

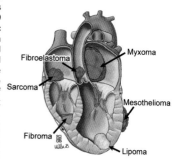

Masses
Myxoma

Cardiac myxomas are single tumors located LA > RA > RV > LV with stalk attachment to the IAS in the atria. The majority possess a smooth, round surface with hemorrhagic and calcific areas. A minority display surface villous fronds which have greater embolic potential.

(A) 2D color compare and (B) 3D Live ME LAX views identify a large LA myxoma prolapsing through the MV causing functional mitral stenosis. (C) xPlane allows rotation around the mass in 2D to further delineate the extent of tumor attachment, surface appearance and anatomical relationships. (D) Alternatively rotating a 3D FV RVOT view shows the IAS attachment and fully demarcates this tumor. Contrast the tumor surface appearances of 2 different large myxomas using 3D Zoom, (E) smooth rounded to, (F) surface villous fronds shown in the surgeon's orientation from the LA.

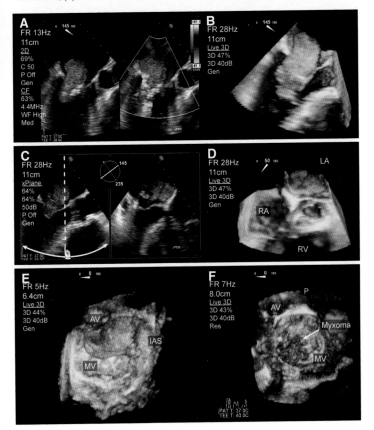

Masses
Papillary Fibroelastoma

These are small lobulated mobile masses located AV > MV > TV, PV, and non-valvular sites. (A) xPlane shows 2D ME AV LAX and LVOT SAX views of a small rounded mobile mass (arrow) in the LVOT. 3D Live (B) unrotated and (C) rotated views show the mass from above as a clearly demarcated lobulated mass without AV involvement and an intact IVS. (D) 3D FV ME dataset rotated to the LVOT side with the LV cropped shows the mass adherent to the IVS below the AV. (E) Exposed through an aortotomy, this unusually located tumor was removed by simple excision.

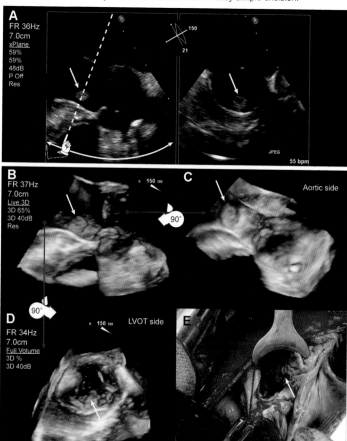

Masses
RV Fibroma

These are typically seen as single, well-demarcated masses located within the ventricles. (A) xPlane shows extensive involvement of the RV free wall and papillary muscle in the ME 4C and modified RVOT views. (B) In this case, 3D Live guided accurate reconstruction of RV morphology to aid complete tumor resection. (C) Surgery involved partial resection and reimplantation of the anterior papillary muscle, RV free wall reconstruction using bovine pericardium and TV repair with an annuloplasty ring. 3D FV views the annuloplasty ring from the (D) side and (E) RA.

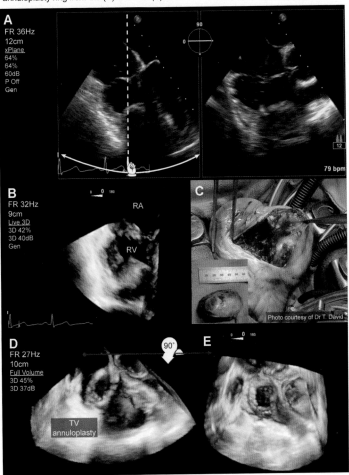

Masses
Lipoma

These are soft lobulated masses located within RA and LV, which occur less frequently than IAS lipomatous hypertrophy. (A) 2D ME AV LAX, (B) 4C views and (D) 3D FV 4C identify a large bright echogenic mass within the LV. (C) 3D FV ME LAX view demonstrates this mass attached to the anterior LV wall and anterolateral papillary muscle without LVOT obstruction or involvement of the MV apparatus. Cropping the 3D FV ME LAX to partly remove the anteroseptal LV wall identifies the point of attachment. (E) A zoomed rotation of the 3D FV ME LAX view shows the mass from the apical LV (arrow) with the MV and AV positioned superiorly. This mass was removed by primary resection without creating new mitral regurgitation.

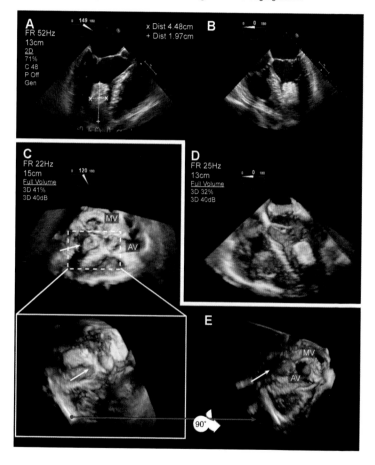

Masses
Cardiac Metastases

These are the largest group of cardiac malignancies involving either the pericardium and or the myocardium.

Two intracardiac melanoma metastases were seen in this patient. (A) xPlane of modified 2D ME 4C and RVOT views identified a RA mass (arrow) adherent to the IAS, AV noncoronary cusp and closely approximated to TV. (B) Rotating a 3D FV ME 5C clearly shows the RA mass attachment and also a PFO. A second metastases is present in the LV. (C) This was poorly visualized using 2D xPlane imaging, although there is a fullness of the apical LV walls. (E) Rotating a 3D FV ME 4C identifies a mass within the posterolateral segment of the LV which did not infiltrate the MV or papillary muscles. Both masses were excised by primary resection with closure of the PFO. The atrial mass is seen in (D) and (F).

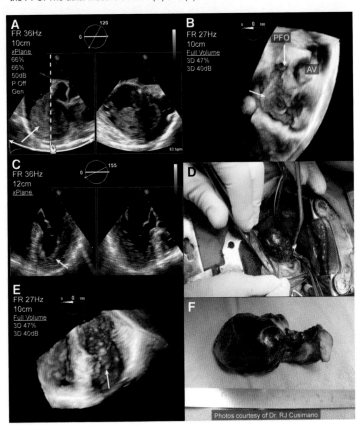

Masses
Anterior Mediastinal Mass

(A) 2D TG SAX and (B) modified ME 2C display a high grade thymoma infiltrating the pericardium. (B) 2D and (C) 3D FV ME 2C clearly show external compression of the LA and main PA (red arrow) by this large thymoma. Intraoperatively, this mass encased the main PA, infiltrated the myocardium and was deemed inoperable.

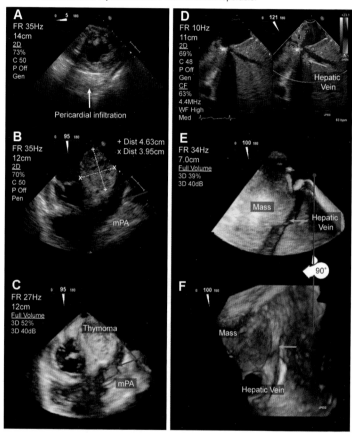

(D) TG IVC 2D color compare and (E) 3D FV images show extension of a renal cell carcinoma into the IVC and compressing the hepatic vein (green arrow). The tumor was located proximal to the RA. (F) Rotating and cropping this 3D FV image shows the mass within the IVC just below the RA. This image shows IVC occlusion with impingement of the hepatic vein. This patient underwent a radical nephrectomy and partial resection of the IVC with this tumor.

Masses
Fibrosarcoma

(A) 2D ME 4C view shows the large sarcoma attached to the LA wall within close proximity of the LUPV. (B) Rotating a 3D FV ME view demonstrates tumor infiltration of the LUPV (arrow) above the LAA with mild narrowing of the RPA. (C,D) The large mass was unattached but prolapsed through the MV causing functional MS and MR. (E) On-line estimation of the mass width is made by overlying a 5 mm grid on a 3D Zoom. (F) This mass showed extensive left lung infiltration with the patient requiring a left pneumonectomy, resection and reconstruction of the LA and MV replacement.

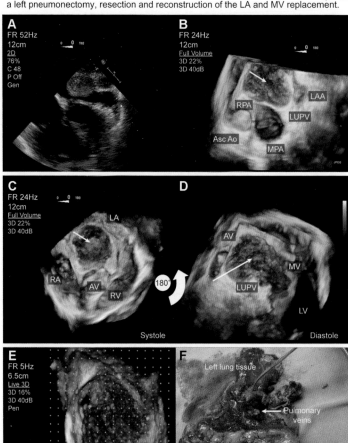

Masses
Angiosarcoma

These are nodular, broad-based masses with a predilection to the RA-IVC junction. This sarcoma commonly demonstrates local pleural and pericardial infiltration.
An angiosarcoma at the RA-IVC junction is seen in (A) 2D modified 4C view centered on the RA and (B) bicaval views. (C) 3D FV image rotated to show the tumor at the RA-IVC junction. (D) 3D Zoom of this area clearly shows the close proximity of the nodular-appearing tumor to the liver. (E) Surgery consisted of tumor resection with part of the IVC and RA under circulatory arrest. (F) The reconstructed IVC and RA junction has laminar color flow in this 3D color Doppler modified bicaval view.

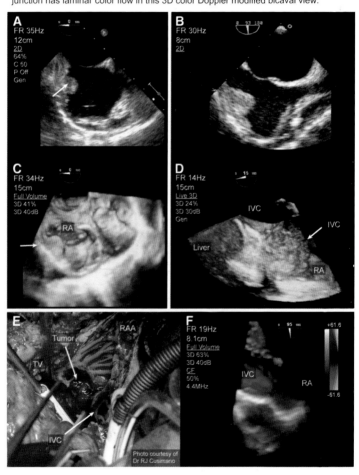

192

Masses
Thrombus

Thrombus appearance ranges from a laminated mural thrombus to soft mobile masses. It is usually located in LAA, LV apex, or attached to catheters, pacer wires, or other masses. A patient presented with RV failure secondary to a pulmonary embolus. (A) 2D ME RVOT view identified a RA thrombus (arrow). (B,C) Live 3D unrotated and rotated RVOT views demonstrate a mobile serpentine mass, traversing the IAS via a PFO and TV (arrow). (D) During surgery a 20 cm thrombus was retrieved from the RA with further clot cleared from the PA.
Another patient presented with rheumatic valve disease requiring MV and TV replacement. An incidental immobile thrombus (arrow) was identified within the LAA on (E) 2D and (F) rotated 3D Live ME 2C views.

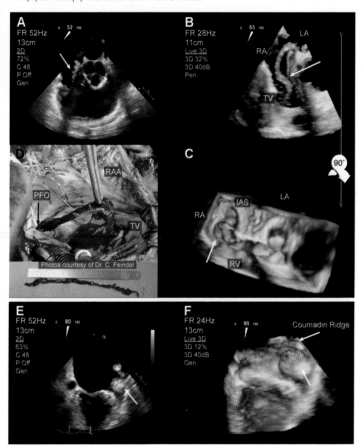

Masses
Endocarditis

Infective Endocarditis
Microbial infection of the endocardial heart surface
3-20% incidence depending on population (native vs prosthetic valves)

Duke Criteria (Source: Durack DT, et al. Am J Med 1994;96:200-9.)
Pathologic criteria: micro-organisms in vegetations
Clinical criteria: (a) 2 major, (b) 1 major + 3 minor, (c) 5 minor
  Major: (1) blood cultures
    (2) echo findings:
      • Vegetations: thickened leaflets, mobile masses move thru the valve during a cardiac cycle
      • New partial valve dehiscence
      • New valvular regurgitation
  Minor: (1) predisposition (see below), (2) fever, (3) vascular, (4) immunologic, (5) microbiologic, (6) echo findings:
      • Valve perforations: jet through leaflet, eccentric
      • Nodular thickening
      • Non-mobile mass

Predisposition for Endocarditis (Source: Circulation 2007; 116:1736-54.)

High Risk (use antibiotics)	Moderate Risk[a]	Low Risk[a]
• Prosthetic valve or repair	• Acquired Valve	• ASD (isolated)
• Previous endocarditis	– Rheumatic disease	• Atheroma
• Heart transplant with cardiac valvulopathy	– Degenerative disease	• ACB
	– MVP with/out MR	• Pacemakers
• Congenital heart	• Congenital Heart	
– Uncorrected cyanotic	– Post repair ASD, VSD,	
– Repair prosthetic material within 6 months	– PDA after 6 months	
	– Complex heart defects	
– Repair with residua at site of prosthetic material	• HOCM	

[a]Antibiotics are no longer recommended

Complications of Endocarditis
• Heart failure: greatest predictor of mortality
• Embolization: mitral > aortic vegetations
• Abscess: hypoechoic area in adjacent tissue without communication with cardiac chamber or vessel, non-pulsatile, no color Doppler flow
• Fistula: abnormal communication between chambers, seen with color Doppler flow
• Pseudoaneurysm of intervalvular fibrosa: echo free area between aortic annulus and base of AMVL, pulsatile with systolic flow from LVOT

What to tell the surgeon:
• Vegetations (location, size, number)
• Valve pathology (pre-existing)
• Valve function (obstruction, regurgitation)
• Complications (abscess, pseudoaneurysm, fistula)

Masses
Mitral Valve Endocarditis

Vegetations form the hallmark of endocarditis
Location frequency in descending order, AV > MV > TV > PV
Usually situated on low pressure side of regurgitant jet, thus

AI → LV side of AV and MV chordate
MR → LA side of MV and LA wall lesions
TR → RA side of TV
VSD → orifice on RV side, TV and PV

Assess for valve obstruction, local complications (abscess, pseudoaneurysm and fistulae)
Assess for risk factors (valve disease, prosthetic valves, shunts, intracardiac cannulae and other masses)

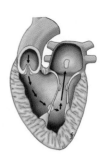

This patient presented with a small mobile vegetation (arrow) adherent to a bioprosthetic MV causing MR as visualized in the (A) 2D color compare ME view. (B) 3D Live modified 4C views during systole and diastole show a sagittal section of the prosthetic valve with prolapse of the mass. (C) 3D Zoom dataset of the entire prosthetic valve is rotated to the (C) surgeon's LA orientation and (D) LV side with the valve struts to show the single mass. There was no associated valve dehiscence or abscess formation. An MV replacement was performed.

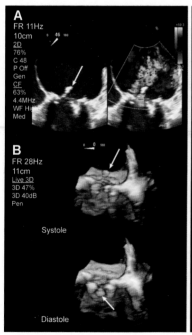

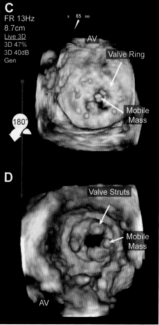

Masses
Aortic Valve Endocarditis

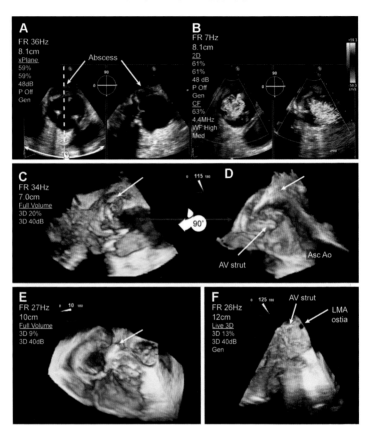

This patient presented with endocarditis after previous bioprosthetic AV and TV replacements. (A) xPlane demonstrates an abscess surrounding the AV bioprosthesis at the native non-and left coronary cusp positions with no color flow (B) which distinguishes it from a pseudoaneurysm. Flow acceleration through the valve is consistent with AV stenosis. (C,D) 3D FV ME AV LAX unrotated and rotated views show extension of this abscess to the intervalvular fibrosa (arrow). (E) Rotated 3D FV ME 4C view demonstrates the TV bioprosthesis with no obvious vegetation but abscess extension into the IAS (arrow). (F) Live 3D AV LAX reveals the inner aortic surface, valve struts, and extensive granulation tissue encompassing the aortic root and left main ostia which still appears patent. This patient underwent homograft replacement of the aorta, reconstruction of the mitral annulus, TVR, patch replacement of the IAS and membranous IVS.

Masses
Endocarditis Pseudoaneurysm

This patient with a previous mechanical MV replacement presented with an intervalvular fibrosa pseudoaneurysm. This is an echo free space (arrow) between the aortic annulus and AMVL base. This dynamic space demonstrates color flow (A) as seen in 2D ME AV LAX color Doppler and expands with systole (B) 2D ME AV SAX. Compare an (C) intraoperative photograph with the (D) 3D Live ME AV SAX and (E) 3D Zoom rotated to show the abscess at the base of the heart.

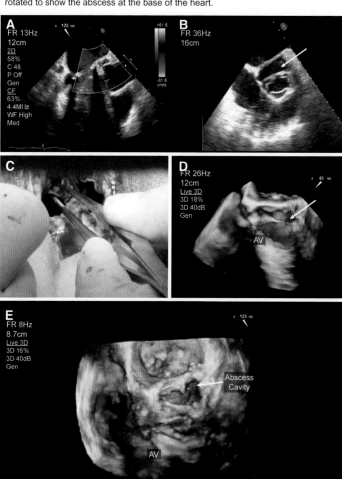

9

Congenital Heart 3D Imaging

	Pages
Congenital Heart Disease	
TEE Segmental Approach	200
Segmental Approach Congenital Heart Disease	201
Congenital Heart Disease Classification	202
IAS 3D Assessment	203–205
Patent Foramen Ovale	206
Atrial Septal Defects	207
Secundum ASD	208
Device Closure	209
Primum ASD	210
Sinus Venosus ASD	211
Ventricular Septal Defect	212–215

A. Vegas et al., *Real-Time Three-Dimensional Transesophageal* 199
Echocardiography, DOI 10.1007/978-1-4614-0665-5_9,
© Springer Science+Business Media, LLC 2012

Congenital Heart Disease
TEE Segmental Approach

1. Determine Cardiac Sidedness (Situs), Depends on Atrial Mass
- Situs (arrangement): solitus (usual), inversus (mirror image), ambiguous (R or L)
- Abdominal situs: solitus (usual), inversus, heterotaxia

2. Determine Cardiac Position
- Based on position in the thorax (dextro/meso/levo-position)
- Based on cardiac apex orientation (dextro/meso/levo-cardia)

3. Identify 3 Segments
- Atrial segments: differentiated by atrial appendage R/L appearance
- Ventricular segments: differentiate as described below
- Arterial segments: PA bifurcated into LPA/RPA, Aorta: coronaries originate

Right Atrium Morphology	Left Atrium Morphology	
Wide necked appendage Extensive pectinate muscles Valves of IVC and coronary sinus	Narrow necked hook-like appendage Smooth walled except for appendage	
	RV	**LV**
Atrioventricular valve	Trileaflet	Bileaflet (unless AMVL cleft)
Leaflet attachment	Septum	Not septal
Annulus location	More apical	More basal
Apex (trabeculations)	Prominent	Less prominent
Moderator band	Present	Absent
Infundibulum	Present	Absent
Ventricular size, shape, and wall thickness do not distinguish R and L Morphologically indeterminate if coarse trabeculations and no interventricular septum (univentricular heart) Tricuspid valve always attaches to RV, mitral valve always to LV		

4. Define the Connections
Atrioventricular connection
- Concordant: RA to RV, LA to LV
- Discordant: RA to LV, LA to RV
- Ambiguous: isomeric
- Double inlet (univentricular) connections 3 possibilities: absent R connection, absent L connection, indeterminate
- Atrioventricular valve morphology: straddling, over-riding, stenotic, regurgitant, dysplastic, imperforate

Ventriculo-arterial connection
2 arterial trunks:
- Concordant: RV to PA, LV to aorta
- Discordant: RV to aorta, LV to PA
- Valve morphology:
  Aortic valve always attaches to aorta
  Pulmonic valve always attaches to PA
- Double outlet: 1 arterial trunk + > ½ other connected to same ventricle

1 arterial trunk:
- Single outlet: truncus arteriosus IV, truncus type I–III
- Outflow tract: muscular (RVOT), fibrous (LVOT)

200

Congenital Heart Disease
Segmental Approach Congenital Heart Disease

1. Determine Cardiac Sidedness (Situs)

Based on position of morphological RA

Situs Solitus
RA lies to right of LA

Situs Inversus
RA lies to left of LA

Situs Ambiguous
Indeterminant/Isomersim

Paired mirror image sets of normally single non identical organs

Right	Left
R Bronchi (x2)	L Bronchi (x2)
R Atria (x2)	L Atria (x2)
No spleen	Polyspleen

Abdominal Situs
Position of major unpaired organs

Solitus   Inversus

Heterotaxia

2. Determine Cardiac Position

Cardiac Position
Based on position in thorax

Dextroposition   Mesoposition   Levoposition

Cardiac Orientation
Base to apex axis

Dextrocardia   Mesocardia   Levocardia

3. Identify 3 Segments

Atrial Segment

Right	Left
• Triangular RAA	• Narrow LAA
• Broad based RAA	• Hook shaped
• Terminal crest	• No terminal crest
• Pectinate muscles	
• (SVC/IVC)	

Ventricular Segment

TV/RV
• Apical SLTV*
• SLTV* chords IVS
• Coarse trabecula
• Moderator band
• Supraventricular crest

*Septal Leaflet Tricuspid Valve

MV/LV
• Fibrous continuity
• No chords to IVS

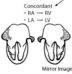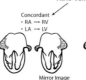

Arterial Segment

Pulmonary Trunk
• Bifurcation to RPA and LPA

Aorta
• Coronary arteries
• Branches to head

4. Define the Connections

Veno-Atrial
• IVC/SVC
• Pulmonary veins

Atrio-Ventricular

Concordant
• RA → RV
• LA → LV

Discordant
• RA → LV
• LA → RV

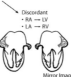

Mirror Image   Mirror Image

Ventriculo-Arterial

Concordant
• RV → PA
• LV → Aorta

Discordant
• RV → Aorta
• LV → PA

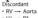

Double Inlet Ventricle
Connection of both AV valves to predominantly one ventricle

Predominant RV
Absent LV

Indeterminate

Predominant LV
Absent RV

Double Outlet Ventricle
Both great arteries arise from predominantly one ventricle

All images courtesy of Willa Bradshaw

Congenital Heart Disease
Congenital Heart Disease Classification

1. Septal defects
   - Atrial septal defects (ASD)
     - secundum, primum, sinus venosus and coronary sinus
   - Ventricular septal defects (VSD)
     - outlet, muscular, inlet and perimembranous
   - Atrioventricular septal defects (AV canal defects)
2. Disorders of mitral valve inflow
   - Anomalous pulmonary venous drainage (total-TAPVD, partial-PAPVD)
   - Cor-Triatriatum
   - Mitral stenosis: supravalvular, parachute
   - Mitral atresia
3. Diseases of left ventricular outflow tract (LVOT)
   - Subaortic, supravalvular stenosis
   - Valvular stenosis
   - Sinus of Valsalva aneurysm
4. Diseases of aorta
   - Patent ductus arteriosus (PDA)
   - Coarctation of the aorta, aortic atresia
   - Truncus arteriosus
   - Vascular anomalies
5. Diseases of tricuspid valve
   - Ebstein's anomaly
   - Tricuspid atresia
6. Diseases of right ventricular outflow tract (RVOT)
   - Subvalvular: Tetralogy of Fallot (TOF)
   - Valvular: stenosis, pulmonic atresia
7. Chambers and valves are in **abnormal** sequence
   - Atrioventricular discordance (corrected transposition)
   - Ventriculo-great arterial discordance (transposition of great vessels)
   - Double-inlet ventricle (with univentricular heart)
   - Double-outlet right and left ventricles

Source: Russell IA, et al. Anesth Analg 2006; 102: 694-723.

3D TEE has been successfully used to assess and enhance our understanding of complex congenital heart disease. Real-time Live 3D has proven to be a useful adjunctive technique to guide percutaneous techniques, for example, ASD closure.

Acyanotic	Cyanotic
VSD	D-TGA
ASD	TAPVD
PDA	Truncus Arteriosus
Pulmonic Stenosis	TOF
Coarctation	Tricuspid Atresia
Ebstein's Anomaly	Univentricle

Congenital Heart Disease
IAS 3D Assessment

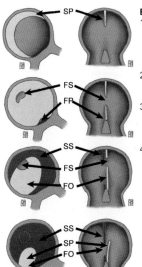

Embryology of the Inter-atrial Septum (IAS)

1. Formation begins with the septum primum (SP) growing down from the dorsocranial wall of the atria towards the endocardial cushions. Above the endocardial cushions is a remaining space called the foramen primum (FP).

2. Perforations appear in the upper SP and form the foramen secundum (FS), allowing for partial reabsorption of the SP.

3. The septum secundum (SS) grows from the ventrocranial wall and covers the FS and FP. The foramen ovale (FO) is an opening which remains and is covered by the SP.

4. The upper septum disappears and the lower portion becomes the valve of the foramen ovale.

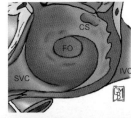

3D TEE of the IAS is difficult with frequent echo dropout due to its location and thin membrane quality. Compare (A) 2D bicaval view with the same views in (B) 3D Live unrotated and rotated down. The latter shows only a portion of the IAS from the LA side. The SVC and IVC are shown draining into the RA.

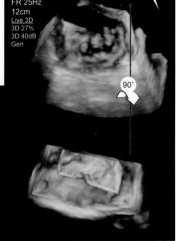

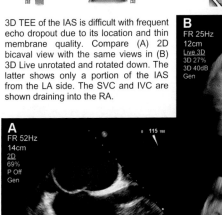

Congenital Heart Disease
IAS 3D Assessment

3D imaging of the IAS can be performed using (A–C) 3D Zoom or (D–I) FV modes. Its thin and mobile structure can create dropout artifacts which need to be distinguished from true septal defects. Images can be rotated to view the defect from the LA or RA side. ASD dimensions are measured by using 3DQ software (Philips Medical Systems). (A) For 3D Zoom position preview boxes to include the entire IAS. (B) The initial unrotated 3D Zoom dataset is shown with a portion of the IAS from the LA perspective. (C) 3D Zoom of IAS acquired at 40° is shown with a more downwards tilt.

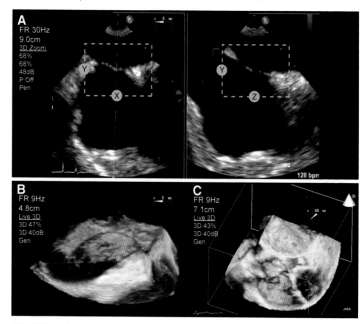

The IAS can be imaged using FV from the ME 4C view (0°) with the IAS positioned in the middle of the display. The initial FV dataset (F) is shown 50% cropped and unrotated. Note the large ascending aorta and position of the SVC which can be referenced to orientate the dataset. (D) Rotating the dataset up by 90° shows the RA side of the IAS with the SVC and superior portion of the IAS at the top of the display. This RA view can be Z-rotated 90° to view it in the surgeon's orientation (E,G) with the SVC to the display left. From image (D) the RA view can also be rotated 180° to the left to show the IAS from the LA. The original FV acquisition (F) can also be rotated downwards 90° to view the IAS from the LA side (H) with the superior portion at the bottom of the display. The LA view of the IAS can be Z-rotated to position the superior portion, SVC and right upper pulmonary vein (RUPV) at the top of the display (I). This patient has a PFO which is easily seen as a cleft-shaped defect in the fossa ovalis from both the RA and LA perspectives.

Source: Saric M et al. J Am Soc Echocardiogr 2010;23:1128-35

Congenital Heart Disease
IAS 3D Assessment

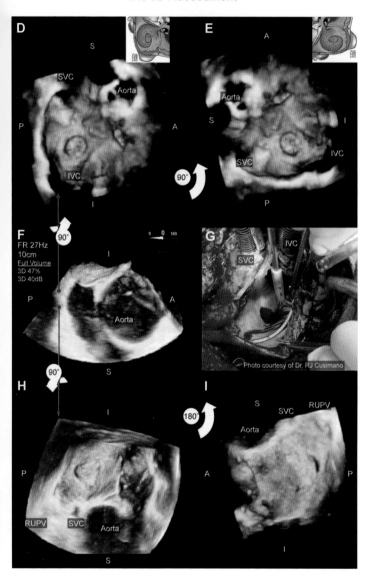

Congenital Heart Disease
Patent Foramen Ovale

(A) PFO is defined by a gap between a flap of the septum secundum and septum primum. (B) There is no absence of tissue (arrow) as shown in an intraoperative photo through the RA in the surgeon's orientation. A PFO shown in (C) 2D ME bicaval color compare view and (D) 3D color Doppler. The gap is best appreciated from a 3D FV acquired from a ME bicaval view and shown from the (E) LA and (F) RA in the surgeon's orientation compare with the surgical photo.

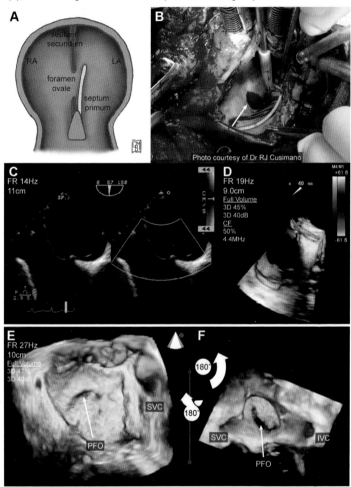

Congenital Heart Disease
Atrial Septal Defects

- Secundum (70%): within fossa ovalis, associated mitral valve prolapse (MVP)
- Primum (20%): inferior septal area, associated ± atrioventricular valve abnormalities (cleft MV), ± endocardial cushion (inlet VSD), aneurysmal IVS
- Sinus venosus (8%): posterior septal area, SVC (superior) or IVC (inferior) type, associated partial anomalous pulmonary venous drainage (PAPVD) from right lung
- Coronary sinus (2%): inferior septal area close to coronary sinus, unroofed coronary sinus drains into LA which also communicates with RA

2D/3D Imaging
- Useful 2D and initial 3D views include ME 4C, RVOT, bicaval
- Assess type, location, size of defect (largest during ventricular systole)
- Volume overload proportional to defect size, results in dilated right side:
  – RA
  – RV, RVH if ↑ PAP, paradoxical motion, and flattening of the IVS
  – Pulmonary artery has increased flow
- Associated lesions: Primum (cleft MV), secundum (MV prolapse), sinus venosus (PAPVD)
- Agitated saline contrast (bubble) study is sensitive in diagnosis of ASD
- Atrial septal aneurysms may have a shunt

2D Color Doppler (3D Color Doppler has limited use)
- Assess laminar versus turbulent flow at reduced Nyquist limit < 30 cm/s and shunt direction

2D Spectral Doppler
- PW continuous flow
- TR is often present due to TV annular dilatation
  – Estimate RVSP (pulmonary hypertension)
- PI if dilated PA, turbulent flow in PA due to ↑ flow
- MR if cleft MV leaflet
- Identify drainage of all 4 pulmonary veins into LA
- Qp/Qs shunt ratios: SV at Qp and SV Qs sites
  – ASD: Qp from PA/Qs from aortic or mitral valve
  – Hemodynamically significant shunt > 1.5:1

What to tell the surgeon:
- Defect type
- Single or multiple defects
- Size of defect
- Identify all 4 pulmonary veins
- RV size and function
- PA size
- RVSP from TR jet
- Agitated saline contrast (bubble) study
- Primum ASD look for cleft MV
- Sinus venosus ASD look for PAPVD
- Persistent shunt post repair

Congenital Heart Disease
Secundum ASD

Secundum ASD displays an absence of tissue within the mid-IAS. It is often oval in shape and varies in size with the cardiac cycle. It is largest during ventricular systole and smallest during atrial systole. Both axes (a and b) are seen in (A) xPlane ME bicaval and (B) 3D Zoom rotated to the LA side. (C) The volume of flow through an ASD is shown using 3D color Doppler in a ME 4C view. A larger ASD involving almost the entire IAS is shown in (D) xPlane and (E) 3D Zoom rotated to the LA side.

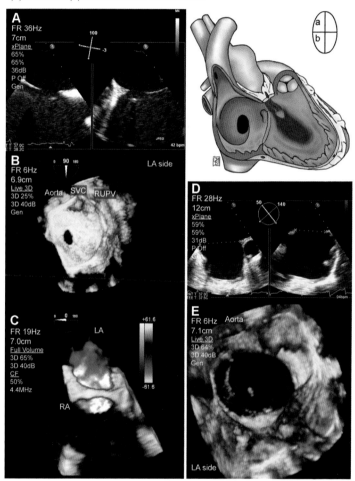

Congenital Heart Disease
Device Closure

These defects are commonly closed percutaneously using as Amplatzer® device which is seen within (A) 3D Zoom orthogonal 2D preview images. A sufficient rim of IAS tissue is required to ensure adequate device placement, aortic rim ≥ 3 mm and other rims > 2 mm. The maximum diameter of the defect should be < 35 mm. 3D Zoom ME modified bicaval views rotated to the (B) LA side and (C) RA side. Post-deployment there is initially some color flow through the device until endothelialization occurs. (D) Color Doppler in xPlane shows incomplete closure of the defect at the IVC border. (E) Maldeployment of a X-shaped " Sideris button" closure device is seen in this 3D Zoom view from the LA.
Source: Jerath A, et al. Eur J Echocardiogr 2010;5:E21.

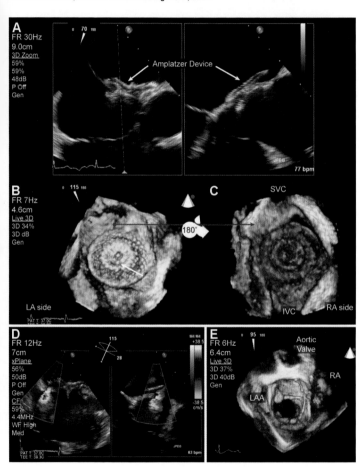

Congenital Heart Disease
Primum ASD

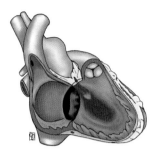

Primum ASD
- Second commonest type of ASD (20%)
- Located in the lower portion of the atrial septum, involves the atrioventricular septum
- Atrioventricular valves are in same plane
- Form of endocardial cushion defect:
  - Partial: primum ASD
  - Complete: primum ASD + inlet VSD + common atrioventricular valve
- Associated defects: cleft MV, subaortic stenosis, double orifice MV, coarctation, PDA, TOF

2D image (ME 4C view)
- Absence of IAS above atrioventricular valves
- Both atrioventricular valves (MV, TV) are in the same plane
- Measure largest gap with and without color
- RA, RV, PA dilated

Color Doppler
- Color turbulent or laminar (unrestricted) flow, usually L → R through defect
- Atrioventricular valve regurgitation: systemic MV → MR, venous TV → TR

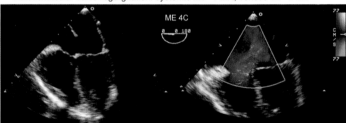

Cleft Mitral Valve
- The cleft is the apposition line between the septal attachments of the superior and inferior bridging leaflets
- Slit-like gap in "anterior leaflet" (arrow in TG SAX view)
- Abnormal chordae to base of IVS (ME AV LAX view)
- Eccentric MR originates at the cleft

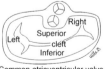
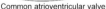

Common atrioventricular valve

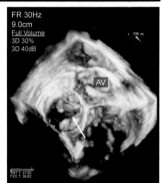

Congenital Heart Disease
Sinus Venosus ASD

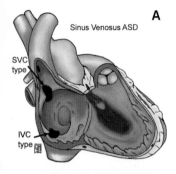

A

(A) **Sinus Venosus ASD** displays an absence of tissue at the RA-SVC or less frequently RA-IVC junction. Anomalous pulmonary venous drainage is a common association with this type of ASD. (B) SVC type shows blue color from LA→RA flow (arrow) with anomalous pulmonary venous drainage (red flow) demonstrated within (B) 2D ME modified bicaval color Doppler and (C) 3D Live views. (D) 3D FV bicaval view rotated to the LA side shows the gap. gap, (E) Importing this dataset into 3DQ (QLab, Philips Medical System) allows measurement of this defect area .

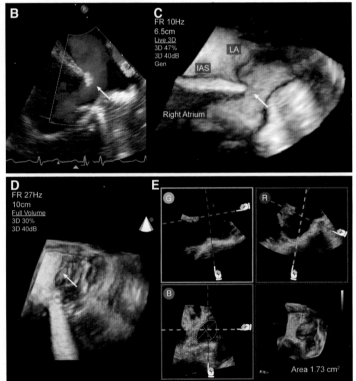

Congenital Heart Disease
Ventricular Septal Defect

Types (may be isolated or part of complex congenital heart disease):
- Perimembranous (80%): below AV and lateral to septal TV leaflet, small
- Muscular: any location in muscular portion of IVS, surrounded by myocardium, multiple, small and difficult to detect by 2D alone
- Inlet (AV canal): posterior to membranous IVS, between TV/MV, associated primum ASD, atrioventricular valve abnormality or complete AV canal defect
- Outlet (5–8%), (supracristal, subarterial, infundibular): RVOT portion above the crista terminalis anterior to membranous septum, below aortic and pulmonic valves

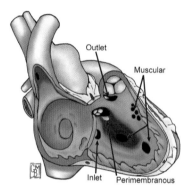

The IVS is best imaged using 3D FV from the midesophageal views with rotation of the image to view the septum from the (A) LV side or (B) RV side.

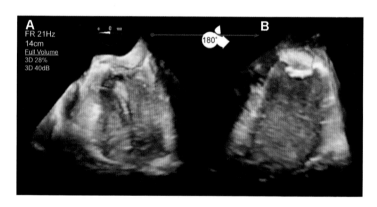

Congenital Heart Disease
Ventricular Septal Defect

2D/3D Imaging
- Useful 2D and initial 3D views are described below
  TTE better then TEE to image IVS
- Assess type, location, size
- Volume overload, dilates left-sided structures and PA:
  - LV size and function (see below)
  - LA dilated from ↑ venous return
  - Pulmonary artery dilatation and ± pulmonary hypertension
- RV less dilated, RVH if ↑ PAP or pressure overload in large VSDs
- IVS aneurysm may be detected, which appears as a " windsock"

2D Color Doppler (3D color Doppler limited use)
- Color helps identify shunt location and direction

2D Spectral Doppler
- CW measure peak systolic pressure gradient between ventricles to classify as
  restricted/unrestricted (see below) and shunt direction (L→R or R→L)
- Estimate RVSP from VSD velocity and systolic BP (SBP), not TR jet
  RVSP = SBP – VSD gradient
- Surgery is recommended if shunt fraction Qp/Qs > 1.5

VSD	Peak Pressure (mmHg)	LA or LV dilatation	Pulmonary Artery Pressures
Restrictive	> 75	no	normal
Mod. restrictive	25–75	↑	↑
Non-restrictive	< 25	↑↑	↑↑

VSD Type	Best Views	Doppler
Muscular	Difficult to 2D image, use color, multiple ME 4C, ME AV LAX, TG SAX	**Color** Flow disturbance on RV side with L to R shunts
Inlet (post to septal TV)	MV and TV in same plane ME 4C	
Perimembranous (A + S TV leaflets) (R + non AV cusps)	LVOT below AV Extend to inlet, outlet, trabecular ME RVOT, 5C, AV LAX or SAX	**Spectral** CW shows high velocity L to R flow in systole
Outlet (below PV)	AV cusp herniation + AI ME RVOT, AV LAX	

What to tell the surgeon:
Pre CPB
- Location (type), size, number
- Shunt direction, peak Pressure gradient
- Associated findings (RVH, RA, PASP)
- Associated pathology: complex congenital, AV cusp
Post CPB
- Residual leak

Congenital Heart Disease
Ventricular Septal Defect

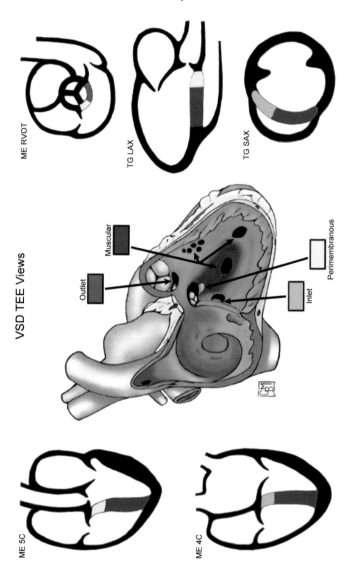

VSD TEE Views

ME RVOT

TG LAX

TG SAX

Muscular

Outlet

Perimembranous

Inlet

ME 5C

ME 4C

Congenital Heart Disease
Ventricular Septal Defect

A VSD (arrow) is demonstrated within the (A) 2D color Xplane, (B) cropped 3D FV ME AV LAX and 3D Zoom ME RVOT views and (C) unrotated and rotated into (E) surgical orientation. Compare (B) with (D) 3D color Doppler ME AV LAX view and (F) surgical orientation of the ME RVOT demonstrating flow across this defect.

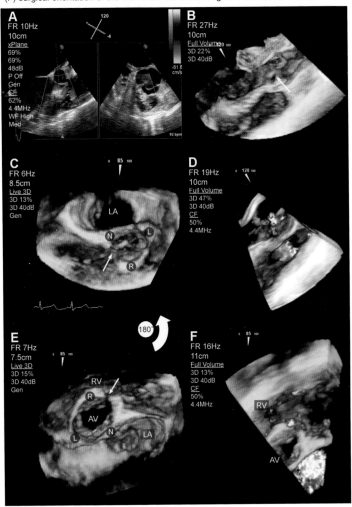

10

Miscellaneous 3D Imaging

A. Vegas et al., *Real-Time Three-Dimensional Transesophageal* 217
Echocardiography, DOI 10.1007/978-1-4614-0665-5_10,
© Springer Science+Business Media, LLC 2012

Pulmonary Vein Anatomy

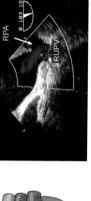

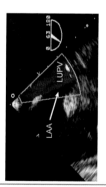

LUPV (ME 60° view)
Easiest pulmonary vein to image. Find left atrial appendage (LAA) in ME 60°, withdraw probe slightly, LUPV lies above (posterolateral) to the LAA and coumadin ridge. Laminar color Doppler flow.

LLPV + LUPV (ME 90° view)
The LLPV is the most difficult pulmonary vein to image. One technique is to keep the LUPV in view and image, then increase the omniplane angle to 90°. The left sided veins appear as an inverted "V".

RUPV (ME 120° view)
The RUPV is easily imaged in the modified ME bicaval view at 110–120°. From the bicaval view increase the omniplane angle to 120°. The RUPV appears in the display near the right pulmonary artery (RPA).

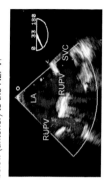

RLPV + RUPV (ME 30° view)
Turn the probe to image the right side of the LA. The RLPV is imaged from 0–30° above (posterior) and perpendicular to the LA. The RUPV is imaged at 30°, below (anterior) to the RLPV.

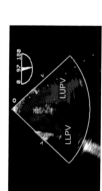

Miscellaneous 3D Images
Pulmonary Veins

The left upper pulmonary vein (LUPV) is easily imaged in the ME view above the left atrial appendage (LAA) in (A) xPlane ME MV 55°. The left lower pulmonary vein (LLPV) is imaged by scanning at 90° and moving the cursor until both veins are imaged simultaneously. The coumadin ridge separates the LAA and LUPV in (B) Live 3D ME 85° viewed from above showing the orifices of the LAA and LUPV and (C) 2D ME view of LAA and LUPV. 3D Zoom of the (D) RUPV in the modified bicaval and (E) orifice of the LUPV in a rotated ME LAA view are shown.

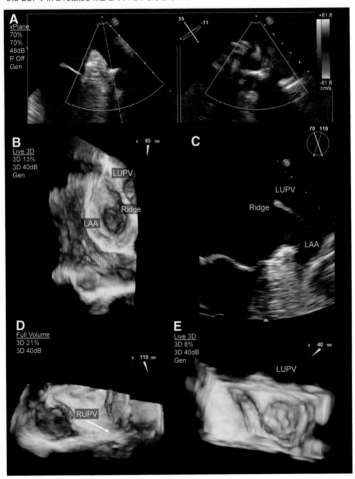

Miscellaneous 3D Images
Pericardial Effusion

- Etiology: inflammatory, infectious, neoplastic, post-MI, trauma, post cardiac surgery
- Location (circumferential, loculated)
  - Pericardial effusions surround the heart (4C, bicaval, TG)
  - Pleural effusions lie posterolateral to descending aorta (desc aorta SAX view)
  - Loculated effusions: post cardiac surgery, inflammatory, metastatic disease
- Echo free stripe between visceral and parietal pericardium
  - Anterior effusion imaged in ME views Posterior effusion in TG view
  - ↓ Echo gain setting to identify pericardial interface (brightest reflector)
  - Isolated anterior echo free space may be an epicardial fat pad
  - Fibrin strands in long-standing effusions or from metastases
  - Thrombus may appear as echogenic soft tissue
- Size
  - Small < 1.0 cm
  - Moderate 1–2 cm
  - Large > 2 cm

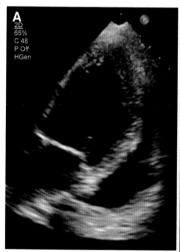

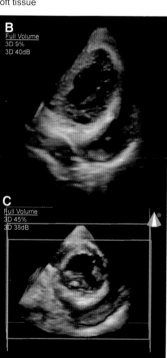

Patient with moderate sized pericardial effusion around lateral portion of LV in TTE (A) 2C apical, (B) FV 2C and (C) FV parasternal SAX.

Miscellaneous 3D Images
Pleural Effusion

Pleural effusions appear as echolucent spaces and are described as claw shaped.
Left pleural effusion appears as echolucent region below the descending aorta.
Right pleural effusion appears as echolucent shape above the liver.
Patient with small left pleural effusion (A) xPlane at 0° and 90° and (B) Live 3D ME
Desc Aorta SAX. (C) Patient with large right pleural effusion 2D ME view.

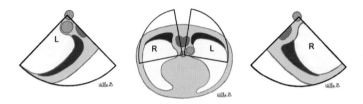

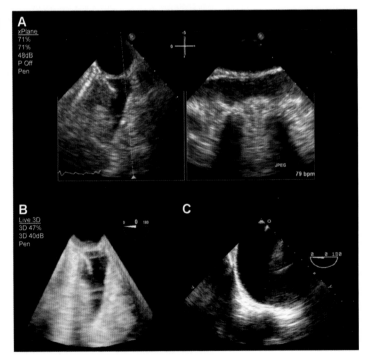

Miscellaneous 3D Images
Ventricular Assist Devices

Ventricular Assist Devices (LVAD, RVAD)

Mechanical ventricular assist devices are used to support the LV (LVAD), RV (RVAD), or both ventricles (BiVAD). They rely on an inflow cannula into the device (outflow from patient) typically placed in the supported ventricle (RVAD or LVAD) or atrium (RA for RVAD). The outflow cannula from the device (inflow into the patient) is placed in the aorta (LVAD) or PA (RVAD). These devices can function as a bridge to transplant and destination therapy.

A) Pulsatile VADs
(HeartMate XVE, Novacor, Thoratec)

The pump with valves provides asynchronous (to native heart) positive displacement of blood into the patient's systemic circulation. In the implanted LVAD, the cannulae and device are both internal, but the power source cable is external. For biventricular support or with smaller patients, both the cannula and devices are extracorporeal.

B) Continuous Axial Flow VADs
(HeartMate II, Jarvik FlowMaker, MicroMed DeBakey)

These devices have replaced pulsatile VADs as the favored devices. These are axial flow devices that use a propeller screw type design, rotating at rapid rates to push blood continuously forward. They are small, totally implantable and durable with a simple valveless design. The DeBakey VAD and HeartMate II (HM II) use typical inflow and outflow cannulae with the axial pump implanted in the thorax. The impeller in the Jarvik 2000 device is implanted directly in the LV apex with the outflow conduit in the descending aorta (left thoracotomy) or ascending aorta (sternotomy). The Debakey and Jarvik devices can support either the R, L, or both ventricles, while the HM II only supports the LV.

C) Continuous Centrifugal Flow VADs (CVAD)
(DuraHeart, HeartWare, Levacor, VentrAssist)

These are considered third generation VAD devices that are small and totally implantable. Some have a relatively short attachment to the LV making them ideal for implantation within the thoracic cavity. An aortic cannula connects device outflow to the aorta. They provide continuous flow by a suspended impeller using centrifugal force. Blood flow enters the device at right angles to its exit.

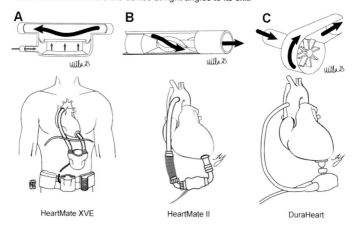

| A | B | C |

| HeartMate XVE | HeartMate II | DuraHeart |

Miscellaneous 3D Images
Ventricular Assist Devices

Ventricular Assist Devices (LVAD, RVAD)
TEE SCA category 2 indication
Pre CPB
Absolute Indications
1. LV and RV function and size
   - RV function determines LVAD filling
2. PFO or ASD
   - Post LVAD hypoxemia R→L shunt
   - Paradoxical emboli
3. Aortic Insufficiency
   - LVAD loop→poor systemic perfusion
Pre-existing conditions
- Intra-cavitary thrombus
- Aortic atheroma
- Tricuspid regurgitation
- Mitral regurgitation/stenosis

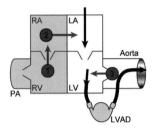

Source: Chumnanvej S, et al.
Anesth Analg 2007;106:583-401.

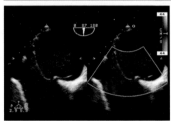

Patent Foramen Ovale (PFO)
- May be difficult to detect as
  - LAP > RAP
  - septum bowed to right/immobile
- Valsalva will increase RAP
  - Color Doppler ± Valsalva
  - Bubble study ± Valsalva
- Presence of a PFO requires closure
- Recheck for PFO post CPB

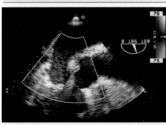

Aortic Insufficiency (AI)
- Underestimate AI severity pre CPB as have reduced transaortic valve gradient from low aortic pressure - high LVEDP.
- Can check AI on CPB (shown) as have high aortic pressure like LVAD flow
- LV vent drain > 1.5 L/min is significant
- Repair or replace AV if moderate to severe AI

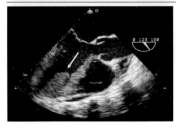

Intra-cavitary Thrombus
- Smoke indicates low flow in the ventricles, atria, aorta
- Presence of LAA clot requires ligation of LAA
- LV clot (arrow) requires careful removal as it may occlude cannula or systemically embolize

223

Miscellaneous 3D Images
Ventricular Assist Devices

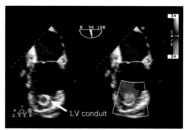

LV Apical Cannula
- Device inflow, patient outflow
- Positioned away from IVS + LV walls, towards MV, see in 2 orthogonal views
- Color: laminar unidirectional flow
- Spectral Doppler (PW or CW):
  - Pulsatile: discrete, < 2.3 m/s
  - Continuous: not to baseline (arrow) 1.0–2.0 m/s

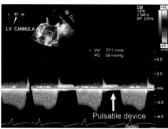

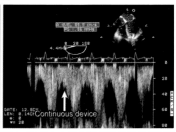

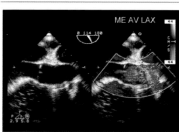

Aortic Cannula
- Device outflow, patient inflow
- Positioned antero-lateral ascending aorta, angulated, pull TEE probe back
- Color: turbulent unidirectional flow
  - Assess aortic insufficiency (AI)
- Spectral Doppler (PW or CW):
  - Pulsatile: discrete, 2.1 m/s, asynchronous to ECG
  - Continuous: not to baseline (arrow) 1.0–2.0 m/s. Pulsatile pattern is LV contraction, synchronous with the ECG.

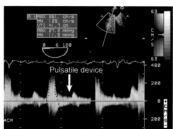

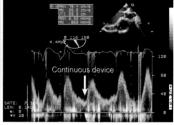

Miscellaneous 3D Images
Ventricular Assist Devices

Patient with dilated cardiomyopathy presented for LVAD implantation. (A) LV reconstruction measured a very low ejection fraction. A thrombus (arrow) was noticed in the LV cavity as displayed by (B) 3D FV ME 4C and (C) 3D Live TG views. (D) The thrombus was removed, a PFO closed, and a HeartWare™ LVAD was implanted. HeartWare™ Ventricular Assist System is an investigational device in the U.S. CE Marking was received for Europe in 2009. (E) The inflow cannula (arrow) at the LV apex is seen with 3D FV. (F) Flow into the inflow cannula is demonstrated by 3D color Doppler. The outflow cannula is visualized in the ascending aorta by (G) xPlane color Doppler and (H) 3D color Doppler.

Source: Estep J et al. J Am Coll Cardiol Img 2010;3:1049-64.

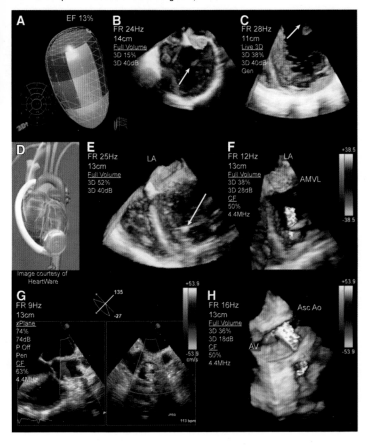

Suggested Readings

1. **Technology**
- Salgo IS: Three-dimensional echocardiographic technology. Cardiol Clin 2007;25:231-9.
- Vegas A and Meineri M. Three-Dimensional Transesophageal Echocardiography Is a Major Advance for Intraoperative Clinical Management of Patients Undergoing Cardiac Surgery: A Core Review. Anesth Analg 2010;110:1548-73.

2. **Basic TEE Views**
- Flachskampf FA, et al. Guideline from the Working Group: Recommendations for Performing Transesophageal Echocardiography. Eur J Echocardiograph 2001;2:8-21.
- Shanewise JS, et al. ASE/SCA Guidelines for performing a comprehensive intraoperative multiplane transesophageal echocardiography examination. Anesth Analg 1999;89:870-84.
- Sugeng L, et al. Live 3-dimensional transesophageal echocardiography initial experience using the fully-sampled matrix array probe. J Am Coll Cardiol 2008;52:446-9.

3. **Native Valves**
- Anyanwu A and Adams D. Etiologic classification of degenerative mitral valve disease: Barlow's disease and fibroelastic deficiency. Semin Thorac Cardiovasc Surg 2007;19:90-96.
- Baumgartner H, et al. Echocardiographic assessment of valve stenosis: EAE/ASE recommendations for clinical practice. J Am Soc Echocardiogr 2009;22:1-23.
- El Khoury G, et al. Functional classification of aortic root/valve abnormalities and their correlation with etiologies and surgical procedures. Curr Opinion Cardiol 2005;20:115-21.
- Eriksson MJ, et al. Mitral annular disjunction in advanced myxomatous mitral valve disease: echocardiographic detection and surgical correction. J Am Soc Echocardiogr 2005;18:1014-22.
- Grewal J, et al. Real-time three-dimensional transesophageal echocardiography in the intraoperative assessment of mitral valve disease. J Am Soc Echocardiogr. 2009;22:34-41.
- Ho SY. Structure and anatomy of the aortic root. Eur J Echocard 2009;10:i3-10.
- Ionasec RI et al. Patient-Specific Modeling and Quantification of the Aortic and Mitral Valves from 4D Cardiac CT and TEE. IEEE Trans. on Medical Imaging 9 (2010);29:1636-51.
- O'Gara P, et al. The Role of Imaging in Chronic Degenerative Mitral Regurgitation. JACC Cardiol Img 2008;1:221-37.
- Omran AS, et al. Intraoperative transesophageal echocardiography accurately predicts mitral valve anatomy and suitability for repair. J Am Soc Echocardiogr 2002;15:950-7.
- Salcedo EE, et al. A framework for systematic characterization of the mitral valve by real-time three-dimensional transesophageal echocardiography. J Am Soc Echocardiogr. 2009;22:1087-1099.
- Sugeng L, et al. Real-time 3-dimensional color Doppler flow of mitral and tricuspid regurgitation: feasibility and initial quantitative comparison with 2-dimensional methods. J Am Soc Echocardiogr 2007;20:1050-7.
- Zoghbi W, et al. Recommendations for evaluation of the severity of native valvular regurgitation with two-dimensional and Doppler echocardiography. J Am Soc Echocardiogr 2003;16:777-802.

4. **Prosthetic Valves, Transcatheter Valves, Valve Repairs**
- Sugeng L, et al. Real-time three-dimensional transesophageal echocardiography in valve disease: comparison with surgical findings and evaluation of prosthetic valves. J Am Soc Echocardiogr 2008;21:1347-54.
- Moss RR, et al. Role of echocardiography in percutaneous aortic valve implantation. JACC Cardiovasc Imaging 2008;1:15-24.
- Zamorano JL, et al. EAE/ASE Recommendations for the Use of Echocardiography in New Transcatheter Interventions for Valvular Heart Disease. J Am Soc Echocardiogr 2011;24:937-65.
- Zoghbi W, et al. Recommendations for evaluation of prosthetic valves with echocardiography and Doppler ultrasound: a report From the ASE Guidelines and Standards Committee and the Task Force on Prosthetic Valves, developed in conjunction with the ACC Cardiovascular Imaging Committee, Cardiac Imaging Committee of the AHA, the European Association of Echocardiography, a registered branch of the ESC, the Japanese Society of Echocardiography and the Canadian Society of Echocardiography, endorsed by the ACC Foundation, AHA, European Association of Echocardiography, a registered branch of the ESC, the Japanese Society of Echocardiography, and Canadian Society of Echocardiography. J Am Soc Echocardiogr 2009; 22:975-1014.

5. **Ventricles**
- Agricola E, et al. Ischemic mitral regurgitation: mechanisms and echocardiographic classification. Eur J Echocardiogr 2008;9:207-21.

Suggested Readings

- Cerqueira M, et al. Standardized myocardial segmentation and nomenclature for tomographic imaging of the heart: a statement for healthcare professionals from the Cardiac Imaging Committee of the Council on Clinical Cardiology of the American Heart Association. Circulation 2002;105:539-42.
- Haddad F, et al. The right ventricle in cardiac surgery, a perioperative perspective: I. Anatomy, physiology, and assessment. Anesth Analg 2009;108:407-21.
- Lang RM, et al. Recommendations for chamber quantification: a report from the American Society of Echocardiography's Guidelines and Standards Committee and the Chamber Quantification Writing Group, developed in conjunction with the European Association of Echocardiography, a branch of the European Society of Cardiology. J Am Soc Echocardiogr. 2005; 18:1440-63.
- Rudski LG, et al. Guidelines for the echocardiographic assessment of the right heart in adults: a report from the American Society of Echocardiography endorsed by the European Association of Echocardiography, a registered branch of the European Society of Cardiology, and the Canadian Society of Echocardiography. J Am Soc Echocardiogr;23:685-713; quiz 86-8.

6. Aorta
- Evangelista A, et al. Echocardiography in aortic diseases: EAE recommendations for clinical practice. Eur J Echocardiogr. 2010;11(8):645-58.
- Glas K, et al. Guidelines for the performance of a comprehensive intraoperative epiaortic ultrasonographic examination: recommendations of the American Society of Echocardiography and the Society of Cardiovascular Anesthesiologists; endorsed by the Society of Thoracic Surgeons. J Am Soc Echocardiogr 2007;11:1227-35.
- Nemes A, et al. Real-time 3-dimensional echocardiographic evaluation of aortic dissection. J Am Soc Echocardiogr 2006;19:108 e1-e3.

8. Variants, Foreign Material, Masses, Endocarditis
- Baddour L, et al. Infective endocarditis: diagnosis, antimicrobial therapy, and management of complications: a statement for healthcare professionals from the Committee on Rheumatic Fever, Endocarditis, and Kawasaki Disease, Council on Cardiovascular Disease in the Young, and the Councils on Clinical Cardiology, Stroke, and Cardiovascular Surgery and Anesthesia, American Heart Association: endorsed by the Infectious Diseases Society of America. Circulation 2005;111:e394-e434.
- Durack DT, et al. New criteria for diagnosis of infective endocarditis: utilization of specific echocardiographic findings. Duke Endocarditis Service. Am J Med 1994;96:200-9.
- Muller S, et al. Value of transesophageal 3D echocardiography as an adjunct to conventional 2D imaging in preoperative evaluation of cardiac masses. Echocardiography 2008;25:624-31.
- Tazelaar HD, et al. Pathology of surgically excised primary cardiac tumors. Mayo Clin Proceed 1992;67:957-65.
- Wilson W, et al. Prevention of infective endocarditis: guidelines from the American Heart Association: a guideline from the American Heart Association Rheumatic Fever, Endocarditis, and Kawasaki Disease Committee, Council on Cardiovascular Disease in the Young, and the Council on Clinical Cardiology, Council on Cardiovascular Surgery and Anesthesia, and the Quality of Care and Outcomes Research Interdisciplinary Working Group. Circulation 2007;116:1736-54.

9. Congenital Heart Disease
- Lodato JA, et al. Feasibility of real-time three-dimensional transoesophageal echocardiography for guidance of percutaneous atrial septal defect closure. Eur J Echocardiogr 2009;10:543-8.
- Russell IA, et al. Congenital heart disease in the adult: a review with internet-accessible transesophageal echocardiographic images. Anesth Analg 2006;102:694-723.
- Saric M, et al. Imaging Atrial Septal Defects by Real –Time Three-Dimensional Transesophageal Echocardiography: Step-by-Step Approach. J Am Soc Echocardiogr 2010;23:1128-35.

10. Miscellaneous 3D Imaging
- Chumnanvej S, et al. Perioperative echocardiographic examination for ventricular assist device implantation. Anesth Analg 2007;106:583-401.
- Estep J, et al. The role of echocardiography and other imaging modalities in patients with Left Ventricular Assist Devices. J Am Coll Cardiol Img 2010;3:1049-64.
- Perk G, et al. Use of real time three-dimensional transesophageal echocardiography in intracardiac catheter based interventions. J Am Soc Echocardiogr 2009;22:865-82.

227

Illustration Credits

Signed Artwork
Gian-Marco Busato: 26-28, 30-49, 55, 56, 68, 80, 100, 101, 108, 116, 120, 136, 140, 158, 160,167,172,175,178,195, 203, 205, 206, 208, 210-212, 214, 218, 220, 222.
Michael Corrin: 2, 3-5,141,154
Willa Bradshaw: 50, 51,124,184, 201, 210, 221, 222
Frances Yeung: 59, 95, 222
Maureen Wood: 54, 96, 176.

Commercial/Physician
TomTec: 74,154,155
Medtronic: 115, 120,128
Edwards Lifesciences: 115,120,123
St Jude Medical: 115,116
HeartWare: 225
H.Houle (Siemens): 86
Dr. Anna Woo, TGH Echolab: 75-77
Gordon Tait for http://pie.med.utoronto.ca/TEE

Surgical Photos
Dr. Tirone David: 91,106,107,110,117,121,169,187.
Dr. Christopher Feindel: 85, 89, 98,105,193
Dr. RJ Cusimano: 186, 189, 191, 192, 205, 206
Dr. Tony Ralph-Edwards: 160,162,164
Dr. Terry Yau: 181

Journals
Vegas A and Meineri M. Anesth Analg 2010; 110:1548-73: pages 2, 8,10,73.
P. Biaggi et al. JACC Cardiovasc Imaging 2011;4:94-7: page 59
Zoghbi W et al. J Am Soc Echocardiogr 2003;16:777-802: pages 61,92,104,111
Baumgartner H, et al. J Am Soc Echocardiogr 2009;22:1-23: pages 66,88,106,111
Lang RM, et al. J Am Soc Echocardiogr 2005;18:1440-63: page 132

A. Vegas et al., *Real-Time Three-Dimensional Transesophageal Echocardiography*, DOI 10.1007/978-1-4614-0665-5,
© Springer Science+Business Media, LLC 2012

Index

Index

Index

Index

234

Printed in the United States of America